It's Not You, It's What Happened to You:

Complex Trauma and Treatment

By

Christine A. Courtois, PhD, ABPP

Psychologist, Independent Practice, Washington, DC

National Clinical Trauma Consultant for Elements Behavioral Health, LLC, and Promises, Malibu

Preface by David Sack, MD

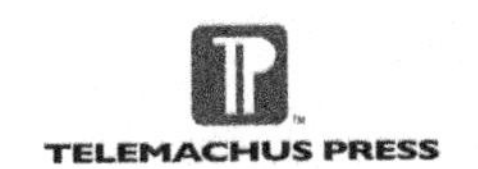

If you purchased this book without a cover you should be aware that this book is stolen property. It was reported as "unsold and destroyed" to the publisher and neither the author nor the publisher has received any payment for this "stripped book."

IT'S NOT YOU, IT'S WHAT HAPPENED TO YOU: COMPLEX TRAUMA AND TREATMENT

Copyright © 2014 Elements Behavioral Health. All rights reserved, including the right to reproduce this book, or portions thereof, in any form. No part of this text may be reproduced, transmitted, downloaded, decompiled, reverse engineered, or stored in or introduced into any information storage and retrieval system, in any form or by any means, whether electronic or mechanical without the express written permission of the author. The scanning, uploading, and distribution of this book via the Internet or via any other means without the permission of the publisher is illegal and punishable by law. Please purchase only authorized electronic editions and do not participate in or encourage electronic piracy of copyrighted materials.

The publisher does not have any control over and does not assume any responsibility for author or third-party websites or their content.

Cover designed by Telemachus Press, LLC

Cover art:
Copyright © Elements Behavioral Health

Published by Telemachus Press, LLC
http://www.telemachuspress.com

Visit the author website:
http://drchriscourtois.com/

ISBN: 978-1-941536-54-4 (eBook)
ISBN: 978-1-941536-55-1 (Paperback)

Version 2014.09.25

Printed in the United States of America

10 9 8 7 6 5 4 3 2 1

Table of Contents

It's Not You, It's What Happened to You:

Complex Trauma and Treatment

Preface

by David Sack, MD

Trauma grows from events both dramatic and everyday—a parent's neglect, a spouse's rejection, sexual abuse, the horrors of war—and brings with it the ability to shatter mental health and spark addictions. Yet its power has long been underestimated.

Historically, the treatment community saw trauma as something to forget and move on from as quickly as possible. The less fuss, the better. Even today, those dealing with addictions within support groups may be told that pointing to past trauma to explain current actions is a way of avoiding the necessary work of recovery.

That's changing as an ever-growing body of research helps us understand that trauma is a force to be reckoned with rather than minimized, and that failing to acknowledge and deal with it only extends the suffering.

Trauma-informed approaches are now making their way into addiction treatment programs, but the change has been slow to come. That's primarily because psychology and addiction medicine have developed along different paths. Addiction treatment grew out of recovery communities that saw little value in analyzing the past. Instead, their focus was on taking responsibility for current actions, no matter their source.

In an integrated treatment program that recognizes the trauma, however, understanding the psychological roots of the addiction is seen as critical to recovery. Without this understanding, the negative coping strategies adopted to deal with the trauma—the drinking, the drugs, the harmful behavior—are destined to recur.

With this book, Dr. Christine Courtois shines a light on all we currently know of trauma, tracing the public's and the treatment community's often grudging acceptance of it as a concept, exploring its many manifestations and, ultimately, illuminating paths toward healing. It's a perspective informed by decades of clinical research and study, her contributions to multiple professional trauma associations, her work as a Board Certified Counseling Psychologist, and her experience running one of the first inpatient trauma programs in the US.

For those seeking to navigate the often confusing and contradictory world of trauma treatment, it's an indispensable resource. Readers will learn, for example, of the multiple types of trauma—impersonal, interpersonal, identity, community, cumulative, and more—and how each interrelates. They'll learn of depression and dissociative disorders and of other issues commonly found in trauma's shadow. They'll discover trauma's ability to affect a person even without that person's knowledge, leading that person to act out in destructive ways without understanding why.

Most importantly, readers get a thorough assessment of the latest trauma treatment options and a guide to creating better relationships and a healthier, happier life. With this knowledge, readers will be able to see themselves more clearly, understand their struggles more completely, and take steps to reverse the downward spiral.

Dr. Courtois' book never shies away from its unflinching portrait of how trauma can shape a person's life, but her message is one of hope. While there is no "one size fits all" treatment for the problems caused by traumatic events, people can free themselves emotionally from their powerful psychological consequences. Trauma-informed treatment can also help the sufferer absorb the message so vital to recovery: It's not you; it's what happened to you.

Chapter One
Bringing Trauma into Focus

Historical Perspective

Not so long ago, traumatized people who sought mental health treatment were likely to be viewed with suspicion and even stigmatized for both their trauma history and their symptoms. This was especially the case if they disclosed a lengthy history and if they exhibited or alleged post-traumatic distress as a reason for their present-day problems and behaviors. Hence, treatment usually did not focus on their trauma or even take it into consideration. Instead, therapists looked at their symptoms, problem behaviors (including addictions), genetics, and/or personality structure. As a result, treatment methods typically addressed one or more of the following:

- Uncovering and resolving the "unconscious conflicts" and "defensive operations" that were thought to be at the root of clients' distress

- Treating clients with "hysterical" or "borderline" symptoms as having major personality problems, with a negative prognosis for improvement
- Strengthening clients' psychological mettle (the "pull yourself up by your bootstraps" approach), to the exclusion of other approaches
- Teaching clients to suppress, deny, or otherwise avoid thinking about past traumas in an attempt to keep those traumas from interfering with present-day behavior and functioning (the "just get over it" approach)

In short, therapists, most of whom typically had little training in terms of understanding trauma and treating its wide-ranging effects, tended to avoid dealing with it. Instead, they told clients that they were making too much of it, that they just needed to suck it up, or that they needed to just move on and "put it all behind them." If you're reading this book in an effort to understand more about trauma and its effects, it will likely come as no surprise to you that none of these approaches is particularly successful. In fact, you or a loved one may have received one or more of these responses in treatment or elsewhere, leaving you without resolution and with little or no hope.

Amazingly, it took the Vietnam War and various social movements of the time (Civil Rights, Women's Liberation, Adult Children of Alcoholics, Dysfunctional Family, and others) to push society and the therapeutic community forward in terms of looking at and dealing with trauma. At the time, Vietnam veterans who'd been routinely exposed to the stressful horrors of combat were returning home with a variety of deep psychological injuries. The emotional impact of the war on these soldiers was both undeniable and significant—witnessed not just by the soldiers but by their friends and family. At the same time, gender-based violence against females—including spousal violence, violence perpetrated by strangers, and the physical, sexual, and emotional abuse of children—entered public consciousness as never before. Meanwhile, the Adult Children of Alcoholics movement focused attention on the long-term effects of parental neglect and abuse, both of which are common in households where parents or others are addicted. Race-based inequities and abuses were also exposed and challenged as never before.

Importantly for that time period (the mid-1960s to the early-1980s), the people impacted by the traumas of war, sexual abuse, spousal abuse, childhood neglect and abuse, and community and racial violence could not be dismissed as merely weak or hysterical, or as confused individuals inventing psychological symptoms for some nebulous secondary gain. Instead, these were red-blooded American soldiers who'd returned from battle incredibly traumatized, people mistreated due to their race and/or gender, children traumatized in their homes by family members, and women who'd been physically and/or sexually assaulted either in the home or by strangers in the community.

In 1980, in response to this increased scientific research and public awareness, the American Psychiatric Association (APA) added a new diagnosis, Posttraumatic Stress Disorder (PTSD), to its *Diagnostic and Statistical Manual of Mental Disorders* (DSM). This new diagnosis identified three primary categories of PTSD symptoms:

1. **Re-experiencing the trauma** in both psychological and physiological ways such as flashbacks, dreams, and nightmares, often in reaction to reminders of the trauma
2. **Numbing of response** as a means of avoiding the pain associated with re-experiencing responses
3. **Hyperarousal**, an uncomfortable state of anxiety, physiological arousal, and associated hyper-vigilance

(Of note: The DSM was revised and updated in 2013 and the diagnosis of PTSD now includes a fourth category of response, **avoidance and cognitive and emotional changes**. It also includes two new sub-types: "Dissociative PTSD" and "Preschool PTSD.")

The inclusion of PTSD as an official diagnosis ushered in a new era in mental health. For the first time, it was officially recognized that psychological symptoms could be due to and caused by real-life traumatic events and experiences rather than some flaw or weakness in the victim's character, the victim's genetic makeup, or some fantasy or wish. It was further recognized that these reactions and symptoms could occur in response to not just current events but past events (even if they occurred in the far distant past). And it was not unusual for some victims to have had multiple and varied episodes of trauma at different points in their lives.

Following the inclusion of PTSD in the DSM, a veritable flood of research on trauma and its impact has been conducted, with numerous treatments developed. Despite this, and even though the idea of past traumas affecting present responses and behaviors has resonated with both mental health professionals and their clients, information about identifying and treating trauma has not, as of now, been widely included in professional training. The unfortunate result is that, even today, many therapists are poorly informed about the link between past (or present) trauma and current mental health problems. They simply don't know how to assess or treat trauma, even when it is directly disclosed by the client. This situation is gradually improving, but traumatized clients still run the risk of not getting a therapist who understands trauma and traumatic stress reactions when they seek treatment.

A Basic Definition of Trauma

Despite the incorporation of PTSD into the diagnostic lexicon more than 30 years ago, a lot of people still don't fully understand what trauma actually is. In fact, even those who've experienced it often don't recognize it. A very basic definition of trauma reads as follows:

> Trauma is any event or experience (including witnessing) that is physically and/or psychologically overwhelming to the exposed individual.

I also like to use an expanded definition:

> Trauma stands apart from normal events in its intensity and impact. It is often sudden, unanticipated, and out of the blue (at least the first time it occurs), making it all the more shocking. (In cases of ongoing trauma, it might no longer be shocking, instead creating enormous anticipatory anxiety for the victim who expects it to reoccur.) Trauma can include exposures and incidents that anyone would identify as overwhelming, such as physical or sexual assault, combat, major accidents, rape, domestic and community violence, child abuse, and terrorist attacks. It can also include exposures and incidents that are less easily identified, such as rejection and humiliation, neglect, abandonment, bullying, and emotional abuse (especially when these occur repeatedly over the course of childhood). Traumas can occur on a one-time basis (as in an accident or a robbery), on a time-limited basis (such as a transportation or weather disaster), or repeatedly to the point of becoming chronic (as in child abuse, human trafficking, and sexual slavery). It is often hard for traumatized individuals to make sense of trauma from an

> everyday perspective since it is so out of the ordinary in most cases. Plus, victims tend to blame themselves—internalizing and personalizing the effects.

These definitions are broad and have both *objective* and *subjective* dimensions, meaning trauma can involve just about any type of adversity or harm, and a person's response is dependent on his or her individualized experience, perspective, and temperament.

Some things easily qualify as trauma. For example, it's hard to imagine a major traffic accident or a train crash not resulting in either physical or emotional stress and/or distress. Nevertheless, a car wreck might be much less traumatic for one person—the guy who drives in demolition derbies for fun, for instance—than for another person, like the new mother who crashed while her infant child was also in the vehicle. In other words, many events and experiences can be traumatic, and what qualifies as highly traumatic for one person may be ho-hum for another.

Basically, trauma is colored by the ways in which a person's physiology was impacted and disrupted by the trauma, how he or she experiences and reacts in the moment, his or her ability (genetic and/or learned) to tolerate and make sense of the experience, his or her personal resilience and hardiness, and the amount and quality of support that he or she receives from loved ones and others after the incident.

Despite the subjective nature of trauma, it is clear that just about everyone has a breakpoint at which traumatic (or potentially traumatic) events or experiences (either single events or traumas that are repetitive and cumulative) cause more than average psychophysiological reactions, resulting in symptoms associated with PTSD—re-experiencing, numbing, hyperarousal, avoidance, cognitive changes, emotional changes, etc.

Unfortunately, trauma is a relatively common occurrence. Most US citizens (80% or more) have been exposed to or personally experienced some type of trauma or potential trauma. For the majority (approximately 75%) of adult trauma survivors, posttraumatic reactions occur in the immediate aftermath but do not progress to PTSD. On the other hand, around 25% of adult trauma survivors do develop PTSD.

Young children, due to their size, dependence on adults, accessibility, and vulnerability, are the most victimized age group, followed by adolescents. And the likelihood of developing PTSD is significantly higher for traumatized children and adolescents than for traumatized adults, especially when the trauma is ongoing with little or no effective response or intervention. In these situations the majority of victims will develop PTSD either at the time or later in life. Unfortunately, trauma in children is not well understood, meaning childhood PTSD is often misdiagnosed as something else—usually as Attention Deficit/Hyperactivity Disorder, Conduct Disorder, or Oppositional Defiant Disorder. Making matters worse is the fact that early-life victimization often results in vulnerability to additional trauma. As such, some individuals have lives marked by ongoing and repeated trauma from childhood forward.

An important point to make here is that trauma, no matter the type or perceived severity, can and often does have not just an immediate impact but lasting effects, some of which might not appear until long after the inciting event. Trauma reactions and symptoms can be ongoing from the time of the trauma or they can disappear for periods, only to resurface later, usually in response to present-day triggers (events, experiences, and even feeling states and physical responses that serve as reminders of the trauma). When this happens, the individual often develops a host of posttraumatic and other symptoms quite suddenly and out of context. In other words, individuals traumatized in the past can experience a wide variety of present-day symptoms and behavioral manifestations, such as recurring fears and nightmares, flashbacks, and other unbidden memories of the trauma that in turn result in ongoing emotional discomfort, severe anxiety, depression, shame, dangerously low self-esteem, inability to form and/or maintain intimate relationships, sexual dysfunction, physical illness, addiction, rage, violence, etc.

Types of Trauma

To better understand trauma, it is useful to parse it into five basic categories:

1. **Impersonal Trauma** occurs randomly due to an "act of God," or simply being in the wrong place at the wrong time. Impersonal trauma includes natural disasters, accidents, and such personal misfortunes as chronic illness, debilitating injuries, and disabilities. While natural disasters and accidents are usually one-time or time-limited, they can sometimes be ongoing and cumulative (think Hurricane Katrina and its aftermath or the effects of the Indonesian tsunami). When impersonal traumas involve chronic illness or disability, they can require ongoing and even lifelong intervention and treatment.
2. **Interpersonal Trauma** is not accidental. Rather, it is deliberately caused and/or committed by one or more people, usually with planning and premeditation. This type of trauma includes all forms of victimization and exploitation, such as abuse and neglect, assault, sexual abuse, community violence, harassment, and the like. When committed by a stranger, this type of trauma is most likely a one-time occurrence. When committed by someone related to or known to the victim, it typically oc-

curs repeatedly. This is due to the relationship between the individuals, the fact that the victim is accessible, and a lack of response or protection on the part of others. An important subgroup of interpersonal trauma is known as attachment (or relational) trauma.

a. **Attachment Trauma (Relational Trauma)** is a form of interpersonal trauma that occurs in relationships where there is primary dependency or a close personal bond, such as a parent-child relationship or a romantic partnership (marriage or the equivalent). Neglect, emotional abuse, physical abuse, sexual abuse, and domestic violence are common forms of attachment trauma. Attachment trauma, especially when it occurs over the course of childhood, has severe developmental consequences that can set the victim up for additional traumatization later in life. This is referred to as *developmental attachment trauma* because it can have a profound impact on a child's development. Attachment trauma can be further dissected into *betrayal trauma, secondary trauma,* and *institutional trauma.*

   i. **Betrayal Trauma** involves the abuse of a relationship or a role for purposes of exploitation. There is often a close relationship between the victim and the perpetrator, such as a parent-child bond or a spousal bond. Domestic violence and various forms of in-the-home child abuse are common forms of betrayal trauma. The difficulty for the victim is that mistreatment occurs in the context of a relationship that fosters needed attachment and dependency and has other, more positive elements that may obscure the true meaning of the abuse. The relationship may be used to obscure or misrepresent abuse, and victims may be "groomed" into relationships where they are later abused and exploited. In these circumstances, the victim and perpetrator often develop what is known as a "trauma bond" as part of their relationship, something that often causes a great deal of later confusion for the victim.

ii. **Secondary Trauma** (also known as the "second injury") occurs when there is insensitivity or a lack of assistance on the part of those whose role requires them to provide assistance, intervention, or protection in the face of danger. Essentially, "insult to injury" occurs when a person or an institution that should provide help does not and/or does additional damage. Take, for instance, a child being bullied at school who is told by a teacher or an administrator to either suck it up or to fight back, with no other assistance or intervention. Rape victims in particular have long complained that insensitive and even degrading treatment by police, criminal justice workers, and medical personnel is often as bad, if not worse, than the actual rape—making the overall experience much more painful.

iii. **Institutional Trauma** refers to lack of response, assistance, protection, or intervention at an institutional level, especially when that institution or agency is charged with providing services to or protecting its members. It also refers to covering up active abuse perpetrated by the institution or its members. This sort of cover-up can involve the scapegoating or punishment of a disclosing or complaining individual (the victim) or those who might be protecting or supporting that person (such as relatives or coworkers). Common examples of institutional trauma include abuse by clergy that is covered up by a church's hierarchy, sexual abuse by coaches that is covered up (i.e., Penn State), and sexual abuse in the military when a cover-up within the chain of command protects the perpetrator(s) at the expense of the victim(s).

3. **Identity Trauma,** as the name implies, has to do with the victim's very identity and personal characteristics. The individual's inherent (and mostly unchangeable) characteristics, such as gender, race, ethnicity, and sexual identity or orientation, are the cause of ongoing discrimination, mistreatment, and violence, even to the point of death. Trauma of this type can occur on a short-term basis or it can be long-lasting, even lifelong.
4. **Community Trauma,** sometimes called *group trauma, historical trauma, colonial trauma,* or *intergenerational trauma,* arises as a direct result of an individual's membership in a particular community or group, such as a family, tribe, ethnic group, religion, or political organization, and the belief systems associated with that group. Not infrequently, community trauma involves conflict and warfare between competing groups, up to and including attempts to eradicate the group (genocide). Trauma of this type can be short-term, or it can last for generations.
5. **Cumulative/Lifelong/Continuous/Complex Trauma** refers to multiple forms of trauma that are repeated, layered, and overlapping. Some individuals have the misfortune of being multiply traumatized throughout their lives.

No matter the type, traumatic events and experiences can objectively range from those that are relatively mild (often identified as "small t") to those that are horrific (often identified as "Large T"). As noted, traumatic events can be accidental or very deliberate. Furthermore, trauma is always subjective. The degree to which a specific trauma impacts an individual depends on the person's experience, genetic makeup, individual temperament and resilience, previous history of trauma and any resultant PTSD, and sometimes even gender (females are more likely than males to develop PTSD), along with the degree of support available. As such, some individuals are more vulnerable to certain types of trauma than others.

The Development and Importance of Attachment Styles

Psychologist John Bowlby developed attachment theory in the 1950s while investigating the reactions of infants and toddlers when they were separated from their parents. Essentially, Bowlby found that, due to their immaturity, infants and young children have extensive need for caregivers (usually parents, though also grandparents, older siblings, nannies, and various others), and they are wired to seek them out in times of distress and danger. In other words, caregivers are relied upon not only for life basics such as food and shelter, but for attention, stimulation, and teaching, along with response and protection when a child feels frightened or insecure. Good caregivers are responsive to the uniqueness of an individual child, supporting the child's positive self-esteem and assisting with emotion identification and regulation.

Caregivers who are consistently available and responsive to a child's needs and development provide a secure base (a "safe haven") where the child can reliably find safety and assistance, and from which the child can comfortably depart, wander, explore, and experience life. Early on, these forays away from the "caregiver comfort zone" are usually quite brief. As children grow older, though, they naturally venture further away, for longer periods of time, eventually becoming separate, secure, and emotionally healthy individuals.

In contrast, caregivers who are absent, impaired/addicted, neglectful, intrusive, anxious, over-demanding, and/or otherwise inconsistent and unpredictable in response create conditions of insecurity. Pervasive insecurity is traumatizing to infants and young children, orienting them toward threat and danger and stunting their ability to explore the world in carefree ways. These children grow up feeling anxious about themselves and those around them, meaning they are insecure and don't feel calm, centered, and self- and other-reliant. They may cope by being excessively dependent on those around them for their self-esteem or by being extremely self-sufficient and mistrustful of others and their intentions.

Following Bowlby's initial research, it has become clear that the level and caliber of attachment experienced in childhood nearly always carries forth into adulthood. People who develop secure attachment bonds early in life usually carry this ability into adulthood, while those who don't very often can't. In other words, early-life attachment disruption and the insecurity it creates can be traumatic, and can significantly affect a person's attachment style, self-esteem, and ability to bond in healthy ways later in life.

In human beings, four primary attachment styles (each of which can have subtypes) have been identified. They are:

- **Secure:** Those with a secure attachment style are confident in the availability and the emotional responsiveness of their caregivers and/or their emotional partners (such as friends or a spouse) and are largely secure in their sense of self. In short, they have a positive self-identity and are able to easily trust others. In times of distress, securely attached children and adults are able to reach out to others for comfort and assistance, and to provide it in turn.

- **Fearful/Avoidant/Dismissive:** Those with a fearful/avoidant/dismissive attachment style anticipate rejection when they reach out to others for comfort and guidance. As a result, they avoid emotional contact and deep attachment in order to keep from getting hurt again, and they often go to extremes of self-sufficiency. Although they appear to be self-sufficient, this is actually not the case; rather, it is a means of self-protection, a way they learned to respond when their needs were not effectively identified or responded to by caregivers.
- **Anxious/Preoccupied:** People with an anxious/preoccupied attachment style do not feel personally secure and are demanding and anxious in their interactions with others. They expect frustration when they reach out to others for comfort and guidance, and they are always on alert for rejection. They are continuously in need of reassurance, relying on others to feel worthy—often causing the very intolerance or rejection they fear.
- **Disorganized:** People with a disorganized attachment style are all over the board with their responses and behaviors. Because their caregivers have been consistently inconsistent and unpredictable and have intermittently mixed good attention with abuse, they fear and don't trust others, and their coping mechanisms mimic their history. Their behavior relating to others, as both children and adults, appears chaotic and contradictory. They may long for closeness with others but push it away because getting close is dangerous rather than comforting. Sometimes they seem psychologically paralyzed, incapable of committing to anything. As adults, they may be anxiety-filled and isolated.

Attachment styles tend to develop very early in life and individuals have little control over their development. Furthermore, attachment styles tend to be relatively stable over the lifespan, meaning those who did not experience secure attachment early in life will most likely struggle with their identity and self-esteem and the ability to develop meaningful and healthy intimate relationships later in life. The good news is that *attachment styles need not be permanently locked in.* With effort and proper guidance, people who were not graced with secure attachment early in life can learn it through therapy and other healthy and healing relationships, creating what is known as "earned security."

Single-Blow Trauma versus Repeat (Chronic) Trauma

Most people tend to think about traumatic events as single-blow occurrences. Most impersonal traumas fall into this category. Natural disasters such as hurricanes, floods, and fires, along with technological disasters like bridge collapses, plane crashes, and chemical spills typically occur once and once only (although there may be many residual events that go along with them). With such events, the severity of trauma symptoms varies widely depending on any number of factors, including the scope of destruction, the individual's degree of exposure, the degree of loss the individual experienced, the public nature of the event, and family/community response. For instance, people in families and communities that pull together after a natural disaster such as a flood tend to experience less trauma than people in families and communities that don't—though individuals within the "pulled together" groups may still be severely traumatized, and vice versa.

Violent crimes and certain other interpersonal traumas also are usually single-blow. Muggings, assaults, rapes, terrorist attacks, and homicides are rarely repeat occurrences. (Homicides never are, though their impact may be very long-lasting to loved ones and friends of the deceased.) Oftentimes these "stranger danger" events impact not only the direct victims of the crime, but family members, witnesses, and even total strangers who merely hear about them. Think about it: If you live in a high-crime neighborhood, it's hard to not be fearful even if you and yours have not directly experienced or witnessed any violence. Terrorist acts—sudden, unexpected occurrences intended to create conditions of fear and anxiety—are actually designed to have this type of widespread impact.

No matter how traumatic single-blow incidents are, repeated interpersonal traumas usually have a greater impact. *Chronic impersonal traumas* such as illness, injury, and disability may require ongoing attention and treatment. *Chronic interpersonal trauma* may begin in early childhood as attachment trauma, which later becomes the foundation upon which other interpersonal traumas are layered. In fact, research tells us that chronic trauma in childhood, especially chronic attachment trauma, often sets the stage for vulnerability to revictimization over the lifespan.

It is possible for chronic attachment trauma to occur even when an individual is not directly victimized. For example, when children witness ongoing domestic violence, sexual abuse, and the like but are not directly attacked themselves, they still suffer emotionally. Usually, the greater a witness's level of attachment to the victim and/or the perpetrator, the more traumatic the event will be. Thus, violence directed by and/or toward a primary attachment figure, such as a father's violence toward a mother, is especially traumatic for most children. Even the mere threat of trauma to a child's loved ones is enough to do lasting damage. So whether kids experience chronic attachment trauma directly or indirectly really doesn't matter; the trauma they experience is profound either way.

Unsurprisingly, chronic trauma arrives in many guises. Some are rather obvious, such as physical abuse, sexual abuse, and violence. Others are less readily apparent, such as non-response or neglect.

In some respects, "neglect has been neglected," meaning it is only recently coming into focus as a recognized form of trauma. Neglect can range from forms that are subtle to those that are not-so-subtle. Most easily spotted is a lack of proper physical care, such as not getting enough to eat, not having decent or clean clothes, not being taken to the doctor when ill or for regular checkups, and the like. Less apparent is emotional and psychosocial neglect, where a person (usually a child but sometimes an adult or an elder) is physically provided for, often amply, but his or her emotional, educational, and social needs are ignored. Though emotional and psychosocial neglect are less easy to spot, they are no less damaging to the victim.

Another form of chronic trauma that can sometimes be difficult to identify (even when it is out in the open) is emotional/psychological abuse. Essentially, this type of abuse involves antipathy and/or intentional cruelty intended to emotionally wound another person, such as when a parent repeatedly tells a child that he or she wishes the child were dead or had never been born, says humiliating or degrading things to or about the child in private or in the presence of others, intentionally deprives the child of basic needs (sleep, food, clothing, etc.), withholds emotional comfort from the child (contact with loved ones or a pet), emotionally blackmails or exploits the child, and more. This sort of calculated withholding and cruelty can actually be more damaging to the victim than less intentional and more impulsive acts of physical or emotional violence.

Family members' substance abuse and addiction can also be traumatic. If nothing else, addicts behave erratically and irresponsibly, in ways that leave the people around them constantly insecure and on-edge, worrying about and anticipating what will happen next. Plus, addicts are more likely than non-addicts to become disinhibited, to lose control of their behavior, and to perpetrate various forms of neglect, verbal abuse, physical abuse, sexual abuse, and domestic violence. In short, children of addicted parents suffer from inconsistency and unpredictability in their parental attachment and their home environment. For them, parents are simultaneously and inconsistently sources of security/protection and threat/danger.

Chronic family violence can create a self-perpetuating cycle. Basically, the abusive family member mistreats others, creating distance and mistrust. He or she may then feel ashamed and may make up for the bad behavior by acting appropriately and lovingly for a period of time (sometimes referred to as the honeymoon phase of the cycle). However, over time, as unresolved feelings and tensions build up, the perpetrator eventually lashes out again. In this way the *cycle of violence and abuse* (and with it attachment insecurity) becomes an ingrained pattern of expected behavior. In such households, lack of personal and interpersonal safety is the norm and uncertainty reigns, leaving everyone constantly on high alert (hyper-vigilant). Hence, even when abuse and neglect occur on a sporadic basis, family members may experience an ongoing state of "anticipatory anxiety."

Other common forms of chronic trauma include (but are not even remotely limited to) the following:

- **Stress Pileup (or Dose-Response):** Studies have found that the higher the dose of trauma, the higher the likelihood of developing PTSD. The trauma dose can involve one primary form of exposure such as combat trauma or result from a variety of exposures that pile up and become chronic and cumulative over time (i.e., attachment trauma, relationship stress, living in a violent neighborhood, living in an addictive household, work stress, financial stress, social stress, etc.)
- **Illness, Injury, and Disability:** Being diagnosed with cancer, learning you are HIV positive, living with chronic

pain, suffering an injury that will never heal, being treated in an ICU, having a disability of any sort, experiencing the effects of a traumatic brain injury or the onset of dementia, and similar situations are now understood to be potentially traumatic and to have traumatic impact. Over time, they create chronic stress that can become debilitating.

- **Grief and Loss:** Losses of many sorts, whether they are sudden or anticipated, can be devastating. Trauma often results in a variety of types of loss, some of which are obvious (i.e., loss of a loved one, loss of a limb) and some of which are not (i.e., loss of personal innocence and self-regard, loss of family safety and a carefree upbringing, loss of good parents and nurturing, loss of religious faith or spiritual belief, etc.)
- **Identity and Cultural Trauma:** These forms of trauma are insidious. If you are a woman born into a society that is strongly misogynistic, every moment of your life is potentially traumatic. The same goes for any minority (race, culture, religion, sexual orientation, sexual identity, etc.) in a society that does not embrace that particular minority or diversity. Dealing with a culturally driven sense of being "less than," in the form of both outright discrimination and more subtle micro-aggressions, can be incredibly distressing and traumatizing, potentially resulting in full-blown PTSD.

What is Complex Trauma?

Complex trauma encompasses multiple and repeated experiences of interpersonal trauma (usually starting in childhood), often becoming chronic. It routinely involves layers of traumatic experience "on top of" or as a consequence of attachment/relational trauma.

Complex trauma survivors are often hyper-aroused and hyper-vigilant on one hand, and numbed and dissociated on the other. Most people with complex trauma histories who enter treatment do so because the many layers of trauma they've experienced in the past are manifesting in the present in ways that are negatively affecting their own lives and quite often the lives of those around them. They often present with multiple, compounded problems.

> *Dean is a 32-year-old highly successful attorney, already on partner-track at his large firm. He enters therapy because he can never seem to maintain an intimate relationship. Though he is initially focused only on his struggles with romance, he admits that his friendships and his business relationships are also mostly short-lived, and even his family ties run hot and cold. After a full assessment, it is clear that Dean has an avoidant/dismissive attachment style. He intellectually and emotionally desires meaningful connections with other people, but he expects rejection, so whenever the possibility of intimacy comes into play his defenses go up. As such, he consistently (albeit unwittingly) engages in patterns of relationship sabotage whenever anyone gets close enough for him to feel emotionally threatened (potentially rejected or abandoned).*
>
> *Unfortunately, whenever Dean feels lonely and/or hopeless about his lack of stable relationships, he numbs out with alcohol and the compulsive use of pornography. He says he comes by these behaviors naturally, as his father was an alcoholic and a womanizer. As for his mother, he says she was alternately loving and then either neglectful or verbally abusive. When Dean was 14 she was diagnosed as bipolar and placed on medication, which lessened but did not eliminate her erratic behavior. During Dean's childhood, nobody ever discussed his mother's issues with him, nor did they discuss his father's heavy drinking and sexual infidelity.*

Dean presents a convoluted yet not uncommon scenario—that of a relatively functional person with many strengths (including high intelligence, a good work ethic, and general resilience and hardiness) along with multi-layered, interwoven patterns of childhood trauma and negative adult behaviors. Complicating matters is the fact that Dean does not believe his childhood was in any way, shape, or form problematic or traumatic, since there were no fires or car wrecks or natural disasters, he wasn't ever bullied, he wasn't sexually abused, his father did not beat him, and his mother loved him as best she could. In fact, he feels that his childhood served to strengthen him, teaching him to deal with adversities and challenges. Nevertheless, it is apparent (based on, if nothing else, the avoidant/dismissive attachment style he demonstrates as an adult) that his childhood was not secure, and that his early-life experiences (his parents' inconsistency and unavailability) underlie many if not all of his destructive adult behaviors, in particular his difficulties with intimacy. In short, Dean's traumatic past is negatively affecting his present-day life.

Not surprisingly, individuals like Dean often deny or minimize the idea that anything bad happened to them. Doing so is perfectly natural, as trauma of this sort ("small t" and cumulative) has not been publicly acknowledged until fairly recently. Additionally, the obvious and understandable reaction to trauma is a desire to avoid and not relive it. Because of this, individuals usually cope by pushing it away, by numbing out with substances and behaviors, by alienating others, and by engaging in various other forms of self-destructive activity—without understanding their motivations for this behavior. Because of this lack of understanding, many traumatized people whose issues manifest later in life (such as Dean) think of themselves and their symptoms as crazy. They don't recognize that their upbringing was lacking and left them without a positive sense of self or needed life-skills, and they don't recognize their problematic behaviors as a natural response to what they experienced. Often these men and women are highly self-critical, blaming themselves for events and circumstances over which they had little or no control. In short, since they don't identify their experiences as trauma, they have no frame of reference for understanding their all too human responses.

It is important to reiterate the idea that response to trauma is subjective. It is colored by the ways in which a particular individual experiences and processes a specific event or series of events. Thus, the alcoholism of Dean's father may or may not have been seriously traumatic for him. The relative depth of pain caused by his dad's drinking will only come out over the course of his therapy. The same can be said for his mother's irrational behavior and inconsistent ability to parent. Nevertheless, his parents' unpredictable behaviors and responses to him are undoubtedly a primary factor in his detached and mistrustful style of relating. It is also clear that his father's womanizing has influenced his perception of women and his tendency to objectify them (through porn use) along with his inability to intimately connect in any sort of lasting way. Essentially, Dean gets into a relationship with a woman, she begins to get too close for his comfort (she "demands" too much emotional vulnerability from him), he starts to feel uncomfortable (smothered and anxious), and then he begins to subconsciously act in ways that are likely to cause a breakup. Afterward, he feels neglected and abandoned, regretting his behavior and yet another failed relationship. Feeling badly, he self-soothes even more than usual with alcohol and porn. Then he feels ashamed, vows to stop and to find a new relationship, and to "make it work" this time. With this, the cycle begins anew. And each time the cycle recurs, another layer of distress is added. Essentially, in an attempt to cope with the unaddressed issues of his childhood, Dean is reliving (or reenacting) it.

Complex Trauma Requires Complex Treatment

Most people who suffer from past trauma that impacted their development and that intrudes into their present-day life in negative ways are dealing with complex rather than single-incident or even single-type trauma. Complicating matters is the fact that many adult manifestations of complex trauma—what are known as "secondary elaborations of the untreated original effects of the trauma," including addiction, chronic depression, severe anxiety, anger management issues, chaotic lifestyles, and the like—require treatment in and of themselves, in addition to treatment for the more classic posttraumatic symptoms. Often these secondary issues must be stabilized first, before the underlying trauma is addressed in any detail. Nevertheless, education regarding the connection of past trauma to present-day behaviors should start early in the treatment process in order to provide a context. This is known as *trauma-informed treatment.* Essentially, this approach recognizes the interconnected nature of trauma disorders and secondary disorders, understanding that if clients don't heal from both, they may not heal from either.

There are numerous approaches and strategies for addressing and de-escalating trauma symptoms and the additional effects of complex trauma in a therapeutic setting. These will be discussed in greater detail later in this book. For now, I will simply say that past traumas need to be looked at (usually in a controlled setting with a supportive person), re-experienced, and emotionally processed to achieve some integration and resolution, to reduce their power, and to reinstate personal control.

Chapter Two
Trauma-Driven Emotional Turmoil

A Basic Understanding of Emotions

Emotions are not exactly the same thing as feelings, although the two concepts are very closely related. Essentially, feelings are *the conscious experience* of emotions. Emotions are often experienced in the body's viscera (the gut) or identified by either facial expression or muscular contraction. By distinguishing between feelings and emotions we can more readily understand the idea of being "out of touch" with one's emotions—something that happens all too frequently with traumatized people. In fact, much of the process of healing from trauma involves identifying, accepting, and feeling (consciously experiencing) the trauma-driven emotions that are embedded in the body and that have long been suppressed, avoided, and/or ignored (in a way to makes them manageable and no longer a source of threat).

Many traumatized individuals, when they first start therapy, are unable to respond to the question, "What are you feeling?" They simply don't know. They know they are feeling something (they may be able to identify a physical sensation somewhere in their body or they may show a facial expression), but they can't identify or name the specific feeling, even when it's something as seemingly straightforward as embarrassed, lonely, or bored. This can be caused by any number of factors, including:

- Early-life inattention to feelings by caregivers (a form of attachment trauma), meaning the individual did not learn as a child how to effectively identify and regulate his or her feelings
- Posttraumatic numbing responses (including dissociation and addiction) as a way to suppress, split off, and not experience uncomfortable or painful feelings
- Associated depression and/or anxiety
- Active avoidance and/or motivated forgetting

Complex trauma survivors often experience various forms of *emotional dysregulation* (an inability to express emotions in modulated ways).

> *Reese grew up the only daughter of two alcoholics. Her father sexually abused her from a very young age and her mother abused her verbally, emotionally, and sometimes physically. With both parents, the abuse grew worse when they drank, and usually* Reese *received that abuse as "punishment" for a real or perceived mistake or shortcoming on her part. Now, as a 25-year-old woman, she is struggling to hold on to a job, to maintain her friendships, and to develop any sort of lasting romantic relationship. She says that she wrestles with intense emotions almost constantly and at times she feels out of control and crazy because of it. She is terrified of being touched by a man, even though she desperately desires emotional and physical intimacy. She also fears criticism from any authority figure. When she does get feedback, no matter how gently offered, she either withdraws completely or flies off the handle. She also has an eating disorder, where she alternately binges and purges.*

> *Unsurprisingly, Reese's unwarranted reactions and idiosyncratic behaviors have resulted in the loss of several jobs and numerous friends and boyfriends, and her eating disorder has caused some serious health issues. When Reese finally enters treatment, she is convinced she's nuts. She has no way of knowing or understanding that her highly emotional and sometimes compulsive responses to certain stressors are learned ways to cope and are actually normal, given the stressors of her childhood.*

Below, some of the more common emotional reactions to trauma (especially complex trauma) are briefly defined and then examined in terms of the ways in which they are apparent with Reese. These emotions are not mutually exclusive. Many survivors of chronic and multiple forms of abuse, like Reese, experience most or all of them at one time or another.

Fear/Terror

Fear is the emotion most closely related to danger, as it is the natural response to the threat of being harmed or overwhelmed (traumatized) either physically or psychologically. In the most severe circumstances (and where threats of harm are routine), fear may reach the level of terror. In extreme and prolonged situations involving terror, emotional and physical shutdown (also known as "freeze" or "collapse") can occur.

Unfortunately, for some victims of trauma, especially when dealing with complex trauma, *fear-conditioning* may occur. In much the same way that Pavlov's dogs were conditioned to expect food whenever they heard a bell ring, trauma survivors may experience a conditioned fear response when reminders of past trauma occur. These triggers can be in any sensory modality: sight, smell, hearing, taste, touch, or any other perception or emotional response. (They can even occur in imagination and dreams.) In Reese's case, she goes on high-alert whenever anyone around her consumes alcohol. She also reacts with fear whenever an authority figure (most notably a boss) looks even slightly cross, especially if that person raises his or her voice.

This type of conditioned emotional response is common with complex trauma survivors. Sometimes it is referred to as the 90/10 response, meaning 90% of a particular emotion (such as fear) comes from past trauma, while 10% comes from an in-the-moment trigger—for Reese, seeing or smelling alcohol and/or observing or interacting with an irritable authority figure. This 90/10 response can occur with all trauma-driven emotions, not just fear.

Anxiety

Whereas fear is a natural response to a real or perceived danger, anxiety is a constant sense that danger lurks at all times around every corner. In other words, anxiety is *ongoing anticipatory fear* and associated hyper-vigilance. With anxiety, threats needn't be seen because they can easily be imagined. Anxiety keeps people in a state of constant readiness, whether that state of being is warranted or not. It is a condition of arousal, where the individual is always expecting the worst. Needless to say, anxiety is exhausting, not just emotionally but physically, creating "wear and tear" on the individual's body and mind. The wear and tear of chronic stress has been found to be related to the development of auto-immune conditions and other physical illnesses. As is the case with fear, almost any cue associated with past trauma can trigger anxiety. Reese's life is fraught with anxiety. Even when work and other parts of her life are going well, she expects that something bad will happen. This is a conditioned response, instilled in her alcoholic household, where nothing was consistent and the unexpected was dangerous.

Panic

Panic is an extreme fear response. A *panic attack* is panic that occurs without a clear triggering event. (If you've ever had a panic attack, you know what a horrible experience it is to be terrified and not know why.) If you're walking down the street and a mugger pulls a gun on you and you freeze or flee, this is panic—an extreme fear response—but not a panic attack. If, however, you have the same response in the middle of an uneventful dinner with friends, this is a panic attack. Unsurprisingly, people who've been exposed to complex trauma are much more likely than others to experience panic attacks. Basically, a terror response that would be appropriate to past traumatizing events can be set off suddenly, without warning, for reasons that are not always clear. One school of thought suggests that panic attacks can be triggered by internal physiological cues like a change in heart-rate, dizziness, or shortness of breath—in essence, physical sensations experienced when the initial trauma occurred.

Sadness

Sadness has been characterized as an emotion triggered by separation and loss. Essentially, sadness signals distress and unhappiness and the need for comfort. Many traumatized people experience agonizing sadness at the time of their trauma and throughout life. Whether they were neglected or more directly abused in the past, they felt alone, uncared for, and unloved—and they frequently feel that way in the present as well. For Reese, anytime she feels abandoned (such as after a breakup or after getting fired from yet another job), she finds herself mired in sadness and isolation, feeling as if she will never be good enough for anyone to love or care about. Even worse, she is unable to reach out to or accept the support of others, no matter how well-intentioned they are. Thus, she is again deprived of the one thing she most needs.

Depression

Depression can be a genetically-based disorder, it can result from all forms of childhood adversity and loss, and it can be the result of grief, prolonged sadness, and/or chronic distress that generates related feelings of hopelessness. Depressed feelings range from mild to crippling. As mentioned above, Reese is generally a sad and depleted person. In truth, she suffers from a significant clinical depression. On a number of occasions she has withdrawn from life and isolated herself—locked the door, turned off the phone, pulled the shades, stayed in bed, and not left the house for days at a time. It is during these times that her eating disorder kicks in, used as a way to cope with her feelings and to soothe herself. In these incredibly dark periods she has ongoing thoughts of killing herself, and in fact she has made several minor attempts. She also engages in occasional bouts of self-injury.

Shame and Guilt

Shame has been identified as having *healthy* and *toxic* forms. Essentially, healthy shame (otherwise known as *guilt*) is the feeling that occurs when a person has done something that goes against his or her values, leaving that person regretting the behavior or feeling badly about it. *Toxic shame* (or just plain *shame*), on the other hand, is the festering internal belief that one is inherently flawed. Basically, guilt is about behavior, the feeling that *I did something bad*, while shame is about the self, the feeling that *I am bad*. The difference between the two is profound. For the most part, guilt can serve as powerful motivation for changing behavior, while shame can keep the individual stuck in a morass of hopelessness. In other words, shame does not encourage or motivate positive change. In fact, the inner life of shame-based individuals continually leaves them feeling unlovable and isolated, and they often behave in keeping with those feelings. Reese is a classic example of a person who has internalized her childhood trauma, believing in her very soul that the abuse she suffered was her fault and that she doesn't deserve anything better in her life. As such, it is hardly a surprise that she feels so badly about herself, constantly expects the worst, and consistently overreacts to even the mildest of present-day slights. She lives a self-fulfilling prophecy.

Alienation

Alienation is shame on steroids. It is the extreme, unshakable feeling of being "less than" and unlike normal people. Alienated individuals are wary of others and mistrustful of their intentions and motives. As such, they go through life emotionally and even physically cut-off, in a constant state of self-protection and defensiveness. They can be highly cynical in their interpersonal and social contacts. As mentioned above, Reese believes to her core that the abuse she suffered was her fault—she should have done something other than what she did to make it stop—and therefore her life is doomed. Unfortunately, she learned early in life that it is dangerous to trust others and that doing so makes her vulnerable to them. This belief keeps her isolated and alone—alienated from herself as well as from others—even when she desperately wants to reach out.

Anger

Anger is a normal reaction to abuse and other forms of mistreatment. Nevertheless, it is often a difficult emotion for survivors of interpersonal trauma. They may deny or suppress it for fear of being out-of-control or becoming like their abuser. Similar to other emotions, anger exists on a continuum of intensity, and it is easier to control and express when it is less intense. It can be used in constructive ways, allowing people to take a stand and to protest mistreatment. Unfortunately, it can also be extremely destructive, especially when it is expressed in directly aggressive and hurtful ways. Anger may also be conveyed through displacement and passive-aggressive behavior where it is misdirected or expressed "sideways" or directed at substitutes (people, places, or things that just happen to be in the vicinity). In therapy, Reese admits that she has lots of displaced anger. Usually, when an authority figure criticizes her, she becomes passive and shuts down. Then, later, her suppressed feelings leak out while she's interacting with a friend or family member. She takes her anger out on them even though the actual source is something or someone else.

Resentment

Resentment is a smoldering, long-term version of anger. Resentment can fester for years, eating away at a person's happiness until nothing is left but seething ill-will. In therapy, Reese admits to resentments against both of her parents, several employers, and numerous ex-boyfriends. She says that sometimes she lays awake at night and relives past traumas they've inflicted, getting either very angry or very frightened as she does this. Although her resentments are justified—especially with regard to her parents—by not resolving them she continues to be trapped in the past in ways that prevent her from healing and growing in the present. The past continues in the present.

Mistrust

Mistrust involves suspicion about and/or lack of confidence, belief, or hope in somebody or something, usually resulting from mistreatment and lack of predictable response. It can develop into the belief that others only act in their own self-interest and with deliberate intent to withhold or harm, rather than in ways that are generous, helpful, and not mean-spirited. Mistrust manifests in Reese's life when she pushes people away inappropriately. For instance, if a coworker is attempting to help her with a difficult project, she feels threatened rather than grateful, unable to trust that person's motivations, and she will often lash out.

Disgust

Disgust is revulsion or loathing directed at the self and/or others. This is yet another typical response to mistreatment and abuse. Sometimes disgust is shame manifested either inwardly or outwardly. In other words, traumatized people who are deeply shame-based can both internalize their shame and project it outward onto others. Reese's disgust is most evident when she is touched by a man, which causes her to feel deep shame about the sexual abuse perpetrated by her father and to push the current man away (either physically or psychologically). She desires intimate contact yet she is repelled by her sexual desires, and she is disgusted by and loathes the person touching her.

Emotions Are Not All Bad

In part, the human stress response and associated emotions evolved as a survival mechanism. For instance, if you're crossing the street and you see a bus hurtling toward you, you are likely to experience fear, which triggers an immediate neurochemical response (the release of adrenaline) and an accompanying physical response (getting out of the way as rapidly as possible). Essentially, when threatened, humans experience strong emotion and react quickly and vigorously. This physiologically-based response, commonly called the fight/flight/freeze response, is automatic and instantaneous, outside of conscious awareness. In this way, emotions are essential to survival.

Emotions also serve as mechanisms for understanding the self. Essentially, emotions trigger a neurochemical reaction as part of a full body-mind physiological response. Although emotions can create problems when they are unmodulated (when they are experienced and/or expressed in all-or-nothing ways, often impulsively and without regard to their effect on others), they are beneficial when they can be experienced and expressed more moderately, with intention, and with the ability to regulate them. At the very least, they are significant to an individual's identity and self-definition, making them extremely important and useful in terms of knowing the self and relating to others in healthy ways.

As we've seen with Reese, the emotions of trauma survivors can and often do run amok. That said, some trauma survivors have the exact opposite experience—a sense of self-estrangement and emotional deadness, identified by the technical term of *alexithymia.* Sometimes these individuals consciously stuff or cut off their emotional responses, fearing that if those emotions (especially fear and anger) are allowed to emerge, the feelings will be so intense that they'll end up going crazy—in the process becoming like their abuser and victimizing others, causing others to reject or abandon them, or committing suicide.

Other times this lack of emotion is an unconscious and involuntary self-protective mechanism. Trauma psychologist Dr. John Briere has labeled this "the pain paradox" because the avoidance mechanism keeps the individual from facing exactly what must be faced if he or she hopes to resolve the problem. Avoidance and other pain suppression mechanisms (including substance abuse and dissociation) are understandable and often work in the short-run, but in the long-run they tend to create and/or prolong posttraumatic problems by interfering with habituation and normalization.

Either way, a primary challenge for most complex trauma survivors involves recognizing, accepting, modulating, communicating about, and even embracing their emotions. The good news is that over time complex trauma survivors can learn to use their emotions in healthy ways—most importantly as a primary means of discerning their needs, their uniqueness, and their identity. In fact, developing this capacity is a primary task in psychotherapy. Essentially, in order to heal, complex trauma survivors must learn how to feel, identify, and healthfully process their emotions. Ways in which this can safely be accomplished are discussed in Chapter Five.

Chapter Three
Other Manifestations of Trauma

Memories

When trauma remains unaddressed and unresolved, survivors may continue to re-experience and relive it—to *remember* it—as though it were happening in the present. They may also (unconsciously and without intent) reenact and recreate it throughout their lives in an attempt to resolve or master it, impacting loved ones and others in the process.

A Brief Primer on Memory

If you think about it, life is lived in large part via memory. For instance, you wake up in the morning and you know where you are and who you are because you remember these things. If you feel a bit groggy, you may decide to make some coffee, and you go about that by remembering where the coffee is, how the coffeemaker operates, and whether you take it with cream and sugar. Even walking to the kitchen so you can make the coffee requires a whole lot of memory. After all, walking is not an innate skill; instead, it must be learned. But most of us don't think much about walking once we've mastered this particular skillset because we *implicitly* or *subconsciously* remember the process on an as-needed basis (unless something happens to short-circuit our memory, such as a stroke or some other catastrophic brain injury). Basically, most of us are able to walk because our brains and our muscles remember how. This is true of our motor skills in general, where we continually rely on the autopilot version of memory.

Other memory processes are a lot more complicated. For starters, our memory networks keep track of sensory, emotional, and semantic inputs.

- **Sensory Memories** involve our five senses: sight, sound, smell, taste, and tactile experience (touch).
- **Emotional Memories** refer to memories with emotional content, whether positive or negative.
- **Semantic Memories** involve ideas and knowledge. In some ways, semantic memories are the "story" that we attach to our sensory and emotional memories.

Most of what we do in daily living involves all three types of memory. Consider the desire for morning coffee discussed above. We wake up and our senses tell us that our vision is blurry and our brain is a little bit slow. Our sensory and emotional memories remind us that when we feel like this, we are unproductive and maybe even a little unpleasant. Then our semantic memory reminds us that a cup of coffee usually makes us feel a lot better, from both a sensory and an emotional perspective, so we decide, based on this, to get out of bed and make a pot of that nice Kona blend we just purchased.

Another useful way to understand memory is to break it down into its *explicit* and *implicit* forms. Explicit memories are remembered consciously and intentionally. If someone asks you what you had for lunch yesterday, you think back to where you were and perhaps who you were with, and you purposefully recreate the scenario in your mind, remembering that you had poached salmon with a side salad and a glass of lemonade. In other words, you *explicitly* remember your lunch. Explicit memory is also referred to as *declarative memory* (because it can be put into words). Sense memories (sights, sounds, tastes, smells, and tactility), verbal knowledge, ability to remember facts, and autobiographical memory (more on this below) are common examples of explicit memory.

Conversely, implicit memory occurs apart from and without conscious awareness. For instance, as I type this sentence my fingers somehow "know" where to go on the keyboard. They don't, of course; instead, my mind is implicitly (and rapidly) remembering how to type and then sending the message through my central nervous system and muscles to my hands. Implicit memory is also called procedural, habit, skill, or muscle memory. Motor skills (such as walking, talking, sitting, and standing) and specialized skills development (as seen in athletes and military personnel) are the result of repetition designed to create implicit memory.

Memory is Not a DVR

Many people believe that memory is like a digital video recorder—capturing every detail of every situation with perfect clarity and permanent accuracy. They think that memory can be called up and replayed exactly as the original experience occurred. Memory researchers have found that this is not the case, and that the way in which a memory is recalled (and the accuracy with which it is recalled) depends on four primary processes: encoding, consolidation, storage, and recall. Some trauma researchers believe that memories of trauma, encoded in conditions of high psychophysiological arousal, are consolidated in different ways and are subject to different forms of storage and recall. In some instances, certain parts of the memory (i.e., the gist of the story) can remain accessible to the individual while other parts (i.e., the more peripheral and/or highly traumatic details and their associated emotions) are split off, though they can return later when traumatic memory is triggered.

Most *autobiographical memories* (personal and chronological memories of lifetime events and experiences) have been found to be relatively accurate though also quite fluid. In other words, autobiographical memories are constantly being built, updated, and even degraded and deleted—a process that can be influenced by many factors. For example, we can incorporate "facts" that others have led us or influenced us to believe, especially when this information is provided by attachment figures or significant others (parents, siblings, spouses), by someone with particular influence (clergy member, boss, coach, military commander), or are societally influenced (information in the media, etc.) Autobiographical memories can also be willfully suppressed or forgotten, influenced by what we (or influential others) don't want to believe or don't want to face about ourselves and our histories. As such, memory researchers must always consider the possibility of false memories created via external suggestions and other influences.

This means that memories of a traumatic event or experience remain fairly constant and accessible for some survivors, while others have little or no recall. People with PTSD often experience the unbidden and intense reemergence of traumatic memories (*hypermnesia*), causing them to vividly re-experience the trauma. Conversely, others with PTSD may experience an inability to recall the trauma (*amnesia*). Sometimes these processes switch back and forth, meaning long-absent memories may reemerge (*recovered memory*) after a period of inaccessibility.

These different possibilities can pose difficulty for people with trauma histories and active PTSD, especially if they have no memory of their traumatic experience or the trauma is in the distant past and disconnected from present-day life. For these individuals, forgotten or dissociated memories of past trauma may turn up unexpectedly, intruding on the present in powerful ways that can be both frightening (reliving/re-experiencing the trauma or aspects of the trauma) and confusing (wondering where this memory came from and if it's real). If you have ever been in this situation, you certainly understand. Wondering if something that you suddenly remember and feel so vividly is real can be crazy-making, to say the least.

Unfortunately, without hard evidence such as witnesses or documentation, there are often no cut-and-dried methods for deciphering what did and did not actually happen. In an attempt to clear up uncertainty, some individuals do detective work, interviewing friends and family members who may have knowledge about or insight into the situation. Even then, the trauma victim is likely to end up with shades of gray, since the memories of others may also be murky, or they might have incentive to not remember, to deny, or to minimize events that occurred or, conversely, to suggest events that did not occur.

Memory and memory accuracy, like trauma, is subjective, influenced by a wide variety of inputs, including (but not limited to) the following:

- **Time:** Autobiographical memory typically begins around age two. Earlier life events tend to not be remembered. (The technical term for this is *infantile amnesia.*) Nevertheless, these experiences are encoded and may return in later life, where they are subject to the individual's interpretation and perspective (and perhaps information from witnesses or documentation). Over time, autobiographical memories are subject to corruption and forgetting.

- **Neurobiology:** Both emotional and physical trauma (and related psychophysiological processes) can interrupt memory formation at any of the four neurobiological stages: encoding, consolidating, storing, and retrieving. For instance, moderate levels of emotional arousal tend to make things memorable in ways that facilitate memory formation, but extreme levels of emotional arousal tend to inhibit it. Also, things like blunt head trauma, traumatic brain injury, stroke, and substance abuse are known to impair memory formation and retrieval. (Have you ever gotten so drunk that you blacked out? If so, you've experienced firsthand an example of substance abuse impairing memory formation.)
- **Social Context:** When families or other social contexts are abusive and enforce the keeping of secrets and/or the silencing of victims, they can substantially undermine the encoding, consolidating, and storing of explicit memory. Betrayal trauma in particular may inhibit the formation of memories, as a means of keeping the relationship with the abuser intact in the interest of attachment and perhaps even survival.
- **Repression:** This is the unconscious, automatic process of avoiding or not thinking about traumatic and other conflicted or aversive events or experiences.
- **Dissociation:** Dissociation is a non-volitional (unintentional) process in which the individual escapes psychologically when there is no physical escape. Dissociation is the alteration of experience, identity, or memory that ought to be integrated. It involves processes of *derealization* ("It's not happening" or "It's not real") and/or *depersonalization* ("It's not happening to me" or "I don't feel anything"). Aspects of personal experience are thus split off (dissociated).

- **Fantasy:** Some people cope with trauma, low self-esteem, shame, and loneliness by escaping into fantasy as a way to avoid and not experience their emotional discomfort. Sometimes a person's fantasy life becomes more real than reality. In such cases, fantasy and reality can become commingled in memory.
- **Forcing:** Suggested or motivated forgetting can interfere with memory, as can suggested or motivated retrieval. Each of these has different outcomes. Material that is real can be made inaccessible, and material that is not real can be suggested and incorporated.

Interestingly, many of the factors that can inhibit the formation of explicit memory do not stop the formation of implicit memory. For instance, specific early-life traumas that occur in infancy and toddlerhood are unlikely to ever be explicitly remembered; however, since they were somatically encoded at the time of their occurrence, they can still affect behaviors later in life through implicit reactions and recall. These implicit memories sometimes provide clues to early-life trauma—clues that can be examined and tested in light of other evidence that might be available. For instance, a person who knows that his or her parents were actively alcoholic during his or her early childhood may not explicitly remember their directly abusive behavior, but from clues he or she may infer mistreatment.

Intrusive Memories (Flashbacks)

Whether past trauma is explicitly or implicitly remembered, its present-day and out-of-context recollection can be incredibly unpleasant and disorienting. This is especially true when memories occur intrusively—unwanted, unwelcome, unbidden. High-intensity intrusive memories that feel as though the trauma is recurring in the present are called *flashbacks*. Their occurrence, seemingly out of the blue, is usually triggered by some sensory or emotional reminder of the traumatic circumstance. Triggers can be something small, indistinct, and seemingly innocuous in the present, such as a sound, a smell, an emotion, or something that resembles the original trauma in some way (a car's backfire that is reminiscent of a gunshot), or even something physiological like a racing heartbeat (from something as innocuous as climbing the stairs).

Flashbacks are sometimes relatively direct replicas of the inciting event (referred to as *flashbulb memories*), remembered and re-experienced in vivid detail. Other times they are much less coherent, blending explicit and implicit memories, emotions, fantasies, and even dreams into a nightmarish, incomprehensible amalgam. The good news is that flashbacks lose their impact when they are managed through the development of grounding skills learned in therapy and through self-help materials, and when they are used for the information they can impart.

The Healing Value of Memory

Healing from past trauma, by necessity, involves remembering traumatic events (usually explicitly but sometimes only implicitly and in somatic forms, without direct recall). Basically, the therapeutic process is a step-by-step, controlled look at past trauma, designed to lower body-based traumatic stress reactions and make them more manageable *before* addressing the trauma. This healing process is based on safety and the building of skills that enable a person to cope with traumatic memories and associated emotions and to interrupt the dissociative process. This is usually a gradual process, though some therapeutic procedures call for more direct exposure to what is most feared and most traumatic.

Whatever means are used, the goal is to access the trauma (especially what has been avoided and/or suppressed in the interest of pain avoidance), and to re-experience and discuss it in a way that makes sense of it and therefore makes it manageable. In short, the therapist helps the client understand that the traumatizing event is in the past, even though the emotional reactions to it in the present are affecting his or her daily life, while also teaching and modeling toleration and management of reactions. This logical look at a very illogical phenomenon in the context of a safe and supportive relationship typically reduces its power and allows the individual to approach rather than avoid traumatic memories, thereby incorporating them with normal event memories. Ultimately, the goal is to disempower the response to trauma and to re-empower the survivor.

Loss of Self and Self-Loathing

Trauma can directly impact a person's sense of self. For example, after a single-event trauma such as a car accident or a weather-related disaster, a victim might same something like, "I don't feel like myself right now." In short, life as it was before the experience has changed, and that change can have a direct and disconcerting impact on the individual. Complex trauma, because it is repeated and/or layered, is usually more damaging, sometimes causing the victim to lose his or her sense of self altogether.

At this point you may be wondering what is meant by the term *self*. It may help to break the concept down into *private self* and *public self*. Your private self is your inner core—how you feel about yourself and how you view yourself. Conversely, your public self is how you are viewed by and known to others. Private self can be further broken down into what are known as *I* and *me*. The "I" portion of your private self is the active, decision-making portion of who you are. The "me" portion of your private self is how you view yourself as an outside observer—the inner narrative you create about your self-concept and self-worth. Interestingly, your "I" is strongly influenced by your "me." In other words, the story you tell yourself about who you are directly influences who you are. Thus, if you think of yourself as helpless and useless, you are likely to actually become helpless and useless, whereas if you think of yourself as powerful and resilient, you are more likely to actually be that way.

For the most part, a person's private self, especially the "me" portion of the private self, develops in childhood in relationship to others. In fact, research shows that during the second year of life toddlers begin attaching words to their self-image, and over the next few years they begin to create a narrative about who they are. Barring neglect, abuse, or other maltreatment, young children develop a fairly positive self-image. It is only when they grow a bit older that they begin to compare themselves to others, often becoming self-aware and self-critical in the process. As children mature, their actual self-image slowly separates from their ideal self-image, and they begin to experience things like shame and pride. When they succeed in various domains of importance (school, sports, friendships, etc.) and when they receive positive reinforcement from people in valued relationships, their self-worth naturally increases, and when they don't, their self-worth diminishes.

Oftentimes, self-worth varies depending on the individual's characteristics and preferences and the arena he or she operates in. For instance, a stereotypical nerd will probably feel better about himself in a science class than on the football field, with the opposite being true for a stereotypical jock. As such, self-worth can vary based on what you are doing and who you are with. If you are with people who like you and/or you are doing something you are good at, your self-worth is likely to be high, and vice versa. Usually a person's self-worth is relatively realistic (perhaps skewing slightly toward the positive). In other words, most people take the good and the bad alike, mix them together, sort them out, and develop a fairly realistic sense of who they are. This is a good thing, as mental and emotional wellbeing is grounded primarily in accurate self-appraisals.

Traumatic experience, especially early-life attachment trauma, is a primary contributor to a skewed sense of self-worth. This can result in the development of a shamed sense of self—the belief that one is inherently flawed, defective, not good enough, and unworthy of love and belonging. Sometimes clients express shame by talking about the "tapes" or "voices" that play on a loop in their head, constantly telling them how awful they are. Others talk about the "shitty committee" that holds meetings between their ears and decides that *everything* is their fault. Still others talk about the gremlins that live in their skulls and scream "No one could possibly love you!" at them 24/7/365. Whenever I hear this or something similar, I know that the origin is most likely trauma-based shame that has negatively skewed the individual's sense of self and self-worth.

As mentioned above, these tapes/voices/committees/gremlins usually develop in early childhood, when individuals are either neglected or abused by one or more attachment figures. Frankly, almost every client I see with significant childhood trauma also has a shame-based sense of self that manifests negatively through a variety of adult behaviors. These individuals walk through life feeling as if they are not good enough, and their negative life experiences serve to reinforce this "fact." For instance, Dean (from the example in Chapter One) and Reese (in Chapter Two) each experienced trauma during childhood and adolescence and they internalized the "messages" of their trauma, turning these messages into a shame-based sense of self. Now, as adults, they've established a pattern of entering into the only sort of relationships they feel they deserve, and their constant struggles in these interactions merely prove and reinforce their shame-filled self-beliefs. Essentially, both Dean and Reese are individuals who've been wounded (traumatized) in ways that cause them to know—not just think, but *know*—that they are unworthy of love, affection, and happiness.

As discussed above, almost any form of trauma can easily be internalized and turned into shame, usually as the traumatized person takes the blame for what occurred. Essentially, abused children (and adults) believe that they deserve whatever abuse they received. If only they could have somehow "done better" or "been better," the mistreatment wouldn't have occurred or it would have stopped. Usually this assumption of blame comes from an internalization of the messages of abuse and a related loss of *self-efficacy*, which is the ability to control a situation and/or to bring about an intended result. Needless to say, a lack of self-efficacy can be highly distressing. Essentially, many traumatized individuals (especially children) attempt to gain control over what is out of their control by deciding that they did something to either cause or not stop it. In other words, they turn around their actual helplessness *by taking blame and responsibility.* In the process, they exonerate the perpetrator. Paradoxically, when the perpetrator is someone of significance to the victim, self-blame rather than other-blame is protective of the relationship. It keeps the victim from being disillusioned and disappointed by someone on whom he or she is reliant.

For the most part, an individual's baseline self-worth and self-concept are relatively consistent over time. We know who we are (or we think they do, anyway) and this self-view doesn't change much on a day-to-day basis. This sense of self-continuity is sometimes called a person's *identity.* Interestingly, we are not born with our identity. Instead, we develop a sense of internal continuity over time, based on messages we and others tell us about ourselves. As such, identity develops primarily in relationship to others and in a social context.

Even though most people's sense of identity is relatively consistent, it is never completely static. Sure, we may see ourselves the same way today as yesterday, or even a month or a year ago, but what about ten years ago? One's sense of identity can and does change—usually very gradually—as part of the normal, healthy, and lifelong physical and emotional maturation process, and also as the result of life events and experiences. Most of the time people don't notice these changes in identity unless they look back across a period of many years.

Trauma, however, has great potential to disrupt personal continuity—including an individual's identity, consciousness, and memories—through a process of dissociation. Many adolescent and adult trauma victims feel as if they have pre- and post-trauma selves, with trauma altering their identity in major (and usually negative) ways. And childhood trauma survivors sometimes say things like, "I'm not the person I might have been," or, "I have a hole in my soul."

Many trauma survivors describe the experience of "leaving their bodies" or "going elsewhere" during traumatic experiences and afterward. This process of *peritraumatic dissociation* takes place when the victim experiences *derealization* ("this is not really happening") and/or *depersonalization* ("this is not happening to me"). This process of dissociation is driven by psychobiological mechanisms set off during the trauma. It is not done consciously or willfully. In other words, self-continuity is spontaneously and temporarily left by the wayside as the person's emotional self-preservation mechanism takes hold. When the individual can later discuss and make sense of the experience, this posttraumatic dissociation can hopefully resolve, restoring the person's continuity and personal integration.

If, however, the traumatic experience is repeated and the detachment mechanism continues to be used and/or there is no way to discuss and process the traumatic event and its impact, dissociation and the resulting lack of integration will persist and eventually become routine. Most of the time, this struggle with self-continuity is directly related to the invalidation or suppression of natural and healthy emotions in order to maintain a needed attachment relationship. In this way the protective mechanism of dissociation is a Catch-22, a double-bind where you're damned if you do and damned if you don't. In short, the splitting off of aspects of reality comes at the price of personal integrity, wreaking havoc on self-continuity.

Healing a damaged sense of self can be a daunting process. Although the damage occurs outside of conscious awareness in response to overwhelming events and experiences, healing is both conscious and intentional. The good news is that trauma survivors are not automatically locked into a life of self-loathing. Instead, they have opportunities to change the way they feel about themselves, and they can do so if they're motivated and willing to work at it. As my colleague Dr. Jon Allen has written, "It's a free country in your own mind." In other words, no matter how badly someone has been neglected or abused in the past, they are not obligated to believe (or act on) their "messages of trauma" in the present.

Troubled Relationships

Just as trauma impacts a person's relationship with self, it impacts relationships with others. In other words, experiences of insecure, abusive, neglectful, and/or disorganized attachment and betrayal lead to not just self-alienation but mistrust of others. As such, it may be useful to briefly recap the nature of early-life attachment, along with the various attachment styles that can develop, as discussed in Chapter One.

As you may recall, Dr. John Bowlby developed a theory of human attachment while investigating the reactions of infants and toddlers when they were separated from their parents. To briefly summarize: children are hardwired to rely on primary caregivers for safety, comfort, and emotional attunement and modulation. Children seek out the "safe haven" of caregivers in times of emotional and/or physical distress, desiring proximity and security. Caregivers who are consistently available and responsive create conditions of *secure attachment,* resulting in children who have a stable sense of identity and who trust and rely on others. Conversely, caregivers who are not consistently available and responsive in healthy ways create conditions of *insecure attachment.*

- Those with a *fearful/avoidant/dismissive attachment style* anticipate rejection and therefore avoid deep emotional connection. They may appear to others to simply be self-sufficient to an extreme degree, but this is merely a way to avoid potential rejection.
- People with an *anxious/preoccupied attachment style* desperately crave reassurance from others, but expect frustration instead. They tend to both seek and fear emotional closeness. They are demanding yet extremely anxious in relationships, clinging but never feeling secure.
- People with a *disorganized attachment style* are all over the board with their behaviors. Their adult style of relating mimics their childhood history of inconsistent and unpredictable attention from caregivers. Their behavior often appears chaotic and contradictory. Sometimes they seem psychologically paralyzed, incapable of committing to anything.

As mentioned in Chapter One, attachment styles developed in childhood tend to persist in adulthood. In other words, people learn and repeat their relationship patterns almost indefinitely. That said, it is possible to change one's attachment style. With effort and proper guidance, people who were not graced with secure attachment as children can learn to securely attach as adults, developing "earned security" of attachment.

Relationship Models: Learn and Repeat

People who develop insecure attachment styles as kids are vulnerable to adult-life revictimization in intimate relationships and elsewhere. Factors that may contribute include:

- An inability to recognize obvious warning signs and dangers
- An expectation of being victimized and/or treated badly
- Living in dangerous families or communities
- Being deferential and compliant rather than assertive in interactions with others
- Being highly dissociative
- Being overly risk-taking and/or aggressive
- Being able to only act out the relational style that is familiar

Until people with insecure attachment styles are able to establish earned security of attachment (through healthy interactions with people who are consistent, reliable, responsive, and trustworthy), they tend to perpetuate the insecure style of relating that is familiar to them. In doing so, they typically partner and associate with people whose relationship patterns both complement and reinforce their own. In these situations, both parties repeat what they have learned over and over without learning that others can truly be trustworthy and reliable.

Commonly repeated relationship issues include (but are not limited to) the following (resulting in many of the emotional reactions identified in Chapter Two):

- **Fear and Mistrust:** People with histories of trauma yearn for intimate connection, but the desired closeness is also what they fear the most. Due to their histories, they suspect and question the good will of other people. Yet, paradoxically and despite these fears and mistrust, they often develop relationships with others. Unfortunately, because they (and usually their partners) are so damaged by trauma, these relationships (now referred to as "dual trauma" couples) tend to play out exactly as they fear, making their prophecies self-fulfilling rather than leading to change.
- **Isolation:** A natural response to interpersonal injury is to develop a fearful/avoidant/dismissive attachment style of staying away from other people as self-protection. The downside of this strategy is that it can create the very vulnerability it is designed to avoid. In other words, isolated individuals don't have a support system to provide perspective and to buffer life's ups and downs. In another variant, isolation is imposed on some victims as a form of control by abusive others. This isolation also keeps them from achieving any degree of closeness or trust.
- **Dependency:** Individuals with an anxious/preoccupied attachment style are often obsessed with the availability and approval of others. They look to others for their sense of self-worth, and they are highly anxious when this approval is not forthcoming or the relationship is threatened in some way. Though their needs are real, their anxiety and their interaction style may interfere with the development of the security they are seeking. In relationships where

addiction is an issue, codependency may develop, with the codependent partner taking care of and protecting the addict in the interest of maintaining the attachment no matter the cost.

- **Helplessness/Victimization:** Trauma is disempowering. As a result, many traumatized individuals have learned to be submissive and deferential in their interactions with others or to express their anger in passive-aggressive ways. Unfortunately, a pattern of being helpless can create a situation of ongoing vulnerability and exploitation.
- **Push-Pull or Approach-Avoid:** Disorganized attachment in particular leads to relational styles that are highly inconsistent. Individuals with disorganized styles tend to attach and detach in unpredictable ways, repeating patterns they learned in childhood and confusing those around them.
- **Control:** A core characteristic of trauma is lack of control. Some survivors cope by controlling as much as possible. They are highly controlling of themselves, their relationships, and their environments. In this way, they protect themselves from ever again feeling powerless and vulnerable.
- **Aggression:** Control sometimes turns to domination and aggression in interactions with others, with the traumatized person switching roles and becoming the aggressor/perpetrator. While this provides an antidote to feeling helpless, it can also perpetuate the cycle of abuse.
- **Seduction:** Patterns of seduction can be related to all forms of insecure attachment. For some people, seduction gives a sense of control/mastery. For others, it brings a feeling of being accepted, validated, and loved. The emotional intensity of seduction can also be used as a way to escape emotional discomfort. (If a person is completely focused on the intensity of romance/sex, he or she can't

focus on the discomfort of shame, depression, anxiety, and the like.) This is especially true with sex and love addicts.

At first glance, one might think that people who've been abused or neglected would try very hard to not become emotionally involved with other abusive and/or neglectful individuals. Unfortunately, the exact opposite often occurs, with victims replaying or reenacting traumatic relationships in a *repetition compulsion.* Essentially, the individual unconsciously plays out what is known, and, in the process of repeating established patterns, he or she attempts to resolve issues from the past (usually without success).

As a young girl Elaine was repeatedly beaten and sexually abused by her alcoholic father. She left home as soon as she could make it on her own. Away from her family, she sought out men she could seduce and dominate; however, most of them were alcoholics who treated her abusively. Nevertheless, she stayed with these men through thick and thin, hoping she could make them "see the light" and cure them of their addiction. Unsurprisingly to an outside observer, they all ultimately left her, usually because they'd gotten arrested and thrown in jail for an extended period or because they found another woman. Following several of these breakups, Elaine got very depressed, and she finally reached out for help. She and her therapist slowly uncovered associations between past and present, recognizing that she was looking for a "good father" in these men, and to cure their (and therefore her father's) alcoholism. Over time, Elaine learned to choose healthier and non-addicted friends as a precursor to having healthier and less abusive dating relationships. She also learned to set boundaries and to have expectations of others as part of her self-assertiveness. In time, she began dating a man who treats her well and who has not had problems with addiction. Her father, now clean and sober for a number of years, recently contacted her to apologize and make amends. She is slowly reconnecting with him, but has not decided whether to forgive him. She wants to see if his actions match his words.

In the example above we see that the effects of trauma on relationships are not an automatic life sentence, but they do need to be attended to and worked on. Simply put, interpersonal trauma—chronic attachment trauma in particular—teaches lessons of betrayal and mistrust and establishes relational patterns that do not allow for intimacy. Learning to reverse these lessons and to engage with trustworthy others sets the stage for more satisfying and reciprocal interactions.

Somatic Effects and Physical Illness

Chronic trauma and resultant PTSD symptoms create a condition of ongoing physiological hyperarousal in anticipation of danger. This creates wear and tear on both the body and the nervous system. The technical term for this is *allostasis*. Over time, allostasis can create serious physical issues impacting all major body systems. For example, too much adrenaline or other stress-related hormones can change the digestive process, potentially resulting in chronic heartburn, a stomach ulcer, or digestive issues. Chronic stress can also lead to muscle tension, headaches (including migraines), heart disease, liver problems, sexual dysfunction, hair loss, skin rashes, and many other physical ailments. Less specific problems related to autoimmune and endocrine dysfunction, including a general sense of malaise or exhaustion for which no specific cause or medical diagnosis can be identified, can also result.

Trauma survivors who've suffered physical injury as a result of their trauma may be especially susceptible to somatic reactions. These individuals may engage in health-risk behaviors either because they don't know better or as a means of self-soothing and/or escaping (through addiction, risk-taking, cutting, burning, etc.), thereby causing even more vulnerability to illness and disease. In essence, behaviors used to cope (smoking, drinking, lack of preventive healthcare, self-injury) may paradoxically create problems in their own right.

Exacerbating matters is the fact that many trauma survivors have phobias about touch, both in general and specifically related to medical care and procedures. Although this is understandable, it often causes them to ignore and/or resist preventive medical care and needed treatment, and to be on "high alert" when interacting with medical personnel. Unfortunately, medical professionals (like most mental health professionals) have typically not been trained to recognize psychological trauma and its many potential manifestations, nor have they been advised about the modifications to standard medical procedures that might be needed when dealing with touch-phobic trauma victims. This lack of training can result in misdiagnosis, mistreatment, and medical care that is less than sensitive to the needs of the patient.

This situation is gradually changing, as "trauma-informed care" is slowly incorporated into medical as well as psychological treatment. At present, it is recommended that trauma survivors make their posttraumatic issues known (without necessarily discussing specifics of the trauma) when they seek medical treatment, asserting their needs and preferences up-front and letting their medical team know that they may have need for more time and explanation regarding medical procedures, more preparation, and more control over the ways in which procedures are applied. Trauma survivors might also benefit from being accompanied by a support person whenever care is sought.

Chapter Four
Common Trauma-Related Conditions and Diagnoses

Assessment of Trauma

As previously discussed, trauma in general and complex trauma in particular have long gone unrecognized and unappreciated as to their profound impact on health and wellbeing. As such, all psychological and medical screening assessments (whether written or verbal) should include questions about past or more recent traumatic events and experiences, asked in behavioral terms like "Did such and such ever happen to you?" and "Have you or any member of your family or group had such and such experience?" Asking about trauma in this very direct way is important because it indicates its significance and gives permission to discuss it. It is also called a *universal precaution*, recognizing that many people do not spontaneously disclose (or even think about disclosing) past trauma unless they are specifically asked. Furthermore, since many trauma survivors don't identify what happened to them as traumatic, asking about specific occurrences or experiences tends to be much more effective than simply asking a general question like "Have you ever been traumatized?"

For formal assessments, therapists typically rely on a combination of interviewing and written or computerized assessment instruments. Some of these formalized tests ask about specific types of traumatic events and experiences, while others gauge aftereffects and symptoms. While assessment is not designed to be stressful, it sometimes can be. Certainly some individuals are relieved to be asked about their trauma histories, but many are not. As such, professionals must maintain awareness that questions about trauma, even when asked with sensitivity, can cause pain and discomfort.

Clinicians should also be aware that traumatized clients don't always give accurate answers. Some of the more common reasons for this include:

- They are not comfortable discussing their trauma.
- They are ashamed of what happened to them.
- They are under threat of retribution if they say anything.
- Disclosure feels disloyal, especially within the family or some other system where loyalty is expected.
- They don't trust anyone in a helping role.
- They don't trust authority figures.
- They don't understand that what happened to them was traumatic.
- They don't think what happened to them is relevant or connected to their current difficulties.
- They can't/don't/won't remember the trauma.

Professionals should not make assumptions about motives regarding nondisclosure. For some traumatized individuals, silence is in the interest of self-protection. For others, a degree of trust is needed before they are able to divulge such sensitive information.

It helps for trauma assessment to be a collaborative effort, beginning with an explanation about how it will be conducted and assurances that the client has control over the process. Furthermore, clients should know that they can ask for clarification if a question is unclear and they can choose to not answer particular questions. The pacing and intensity of questions should be adjusted based on individual needs and concerns. The assessment can be paused or even stopped if it is too stressful. When clients understand that the professional is respectful and attentive and is trying to uncover and understand the issues *with them*, they are more likely to accurately report their experiences and symptoms.

Trauma Doesn't Always Lead to a Disorder

It is important to note that not all trauma results in a diagnosis of PTSD or any other psychological disorder. *For adults, PTSD and other trauma-related disorders are the atypical trauma response.* In fact, the majority of adults experience posttraumatic reactions that resolve in a relatively short period of time (approximately one month) after the traumatic event. As an example, consider an adult with a solid support network and a minimal past trauma history who's involved in a fender-bender after another driver misses a stop sign. That person will likely experience fear, anger, and various other emotions immediately and in the short-term aftermath. He or she might repeatedly tell family and friends about it, getting reassurance in the process. He or she might have bad dreams about car accidents and become anxious whenever a stop sign is approached, hyper-vigilant to the possibility of another accident. After several weeks, however, these reactions generally lessen and the person returns to normal.

For children and adolescents the situation is different. *Young people are much more likely than adults to develop trauma-related disorders, especially when trauma is repeated and no relief or support is available.*

When a trauma-related disorder does develop, it is usually because the individual's coping capacity has been overwhelmed, psychologically and physiologically. When this happens, normal posttraumatic reactions and dissociative processes become *symptoms.* These posttraumatic symptoms can range in severity from those that are relatively mild annoyances to those that are quite severe, sometimes to the point of being agonizing or even life-threatening. They can emerge continuously from the time of the trauma, or they can be sporadic, sometimes emerging in delayed form long after the inciting event. Common trauma-driven disorders include stress disorders, dissociative disorders, addictions, and numerous others.

Stress Disorders

Acute Stress Disorder

Acute stress disorder (ASD) occurs in the immediate aftermath of a traumatic event or experience. In many respects it is similar to PTSD, but it is much shorter in duration, lasting anywhere from three days to a month. ASD symptoms that last longer than a month qualify as PTSD. In addition to the defined timeframe, a diagnosis of ASD requires:

- Exposure to trauma
- Some combination of intrusive memories, negative mood, dissociative symptoms, avoidance, and arousal symptoms (anxiety, hyper-vigilance, etc.)
- Clinically significant distress or impairment in social, occupational, or other important areas of functioning

During periods of ASD, traumatic events can be re-experienced in various ways. Most commonly the individual has recurrent and intrusive recollections of the event triggered by any number of factors (sights, sounds, smells, etc.) As mentioned above, ASD lasting longer than a month meets criteria for PTSD. As such, ASD is typically viewed as a precursor to PTSD.

Posttraumatic Stress Disorder

PTSD has been discussed extensively throughout this book. The diagnostic criteria for PTSD are roughly the same as for ASD, except the symptoms stick around for longer than a month after the trauma, sometimes disappearing and then reappearing many years later. In short, when an individual's physiology and psychology have been disrupted enough to cause symptoms in four primary areas (re-experiencing the trauma through dreams, memories, and flashbacks; avoiding reminders of the trauma; engaging in numbing strategies to deal with painful emotions and related cognitive changes; and experiencing hyperarousal and hyper-vigilance), the diagnosis of PTSD is warranted.

Symptoms of PTSD can be quite debilitating, and they are often accompanied by depression, anxiety, and other reactions that, in and of themselves, can be serious enough to merit separate diagnoses. Plus, people with PTSD sometimes turn to alcohol, drugs, and/or potentially addictive behaviors (gambling, spending, eating, sex, etc.) to cope with the painful psychological and physiological reactions they have when triggered to remember and re-experience past traumas. This use of addictive substances and behaviors can be an effective short-term coping strategy, but over time addiction can result, creating serious problems in its own right.

Complex PTSD

Known colloquially as "PTSD plus," complex PTSD refers to a set of additional responses and symptoms beyond those that make up the PTSD diagnosis. Additional considerations for complex PTSD include the impact on the individual's identity and self-worth, the ability to identify and regulate emotions, and the ability to trust and relate to others in healthy and intimate ways. Complex PTSD can further result in dissociation, physical illness, and a loss of life-meaning, spirituality, and overall life satisfaction. Typically, complex PTSD symptoms do not get recognized as trauma-related, meaning they are often misunderstood and left untreated.

The complex PTSD formulation was created, in part, as an umbrella diagnosis for all of the non-stress disorder reactions that typically accompany complex trauma. Several of these reactions are discussed below. Unfortunately, at the present time complex PTSD is not a free-standing diagnosis in the DSM; rather, it is an associated feature of PTSD. This means that therapists are still required to diagnose both standard PTSD and any secondary disorders such as depression or anxiety if they wish to account for all of the client's co-occurring symptoms and issues.

Dissociative Reactions and Disorders

Psychiatrist Richard Kluft has defined dissociation as taking mental flight when physical flight is impossible. In this sense, it is easy to understand dissociation as a self-protective coping mechanism that occurs when other options are not readily available. Dissociation is especially operational in childhood and adolescence. There are many forms of dissociation, everything from daydreaming to dis-remembering events to complete shifts in identity. Though dissociation is not always the result of trauma, it is clear that trauma is typically an underlying issue. Knowing this, it is hardly surprising that dissociative disorders tend to overlap with PTSD.

Peritraumatic dissociation occurs during and/or immediately after a traumatic experience when an individual enters a state that involves feeling numb, detached (physically and/or mentally), dazed, disoriented, or separated from events as they are happening. *Peritraumatic dissociation is relatively normal and is not considered pathological.* Nevertheless, research shows that peritraumatic dissociation is associated with an increased likelihood of PTSD because, although protective at the time of the trauma, it interferes with processing.

Several dissociative disorders are included in the DSM:

- **Depersonalization/Derealization Disorder:** *Depersonalization* is the experience of being an outside observer with respect to one's thoughts, feelings, sensations, body, or actions (an unreal or absent self, distorted perceptions of time, emotional/physical numbness, etc.) The individual may report thoughts like, "I have no self," or, "This is not me." *Derealization* is the experience of unreality or detachment with respect to surroundings (other individuals are experienced as unreal, life is dream-like/foggy/distorted, etc.) The individual may report thoughts like, "I don't feel my feelings," or, "I know I have thoughts but they don't seem like they're mine."
- **Dissociative Amnesia:** Dissociative amnesia is the inability to recall important personal information, usually of a traumatic or stressful nature, that is too extensive to be explained by ordinary forgetfulness. Often, dissociative amnesia is reversible through extensive therapeutic work. That said, because memories formed in conditions of detachment are by nature somewhat fuzzy, it can't be assumed that all memories can be recovered, or that the memories that are recovered are entirely accurate.

- **Dissociative Amnesia with Dissociative Fugue:** A fugue state is amnesia to an extreme, usually involving sudden, unexpected travel away from one's home or one's work, coupled with an inability to remember one's past, confusion about one's identity, or the development of a new identity. Fugues are usually triggered by extreme stress or trauma.
- **Dissociative Identity Disorder:** Formerly called multiple personality disorder, dissociative identity disorder involves two or more distinct identities that recurrently take control of a person's behavior. Most often, dissociative identity disorder develops in conjunction with severe and prolonged childhood trauma.

Co-Occurring Conditions and Disorders

As mentioned above, posttraumatic disorders are often accompanied by co-occurring psychological and physical disorders. The most common include depression, bipolar disorder, anxiety, and schizophrenia spectrum disorders.

Depression

Trauma is by no means the only potential cause for depression—genetic predisposition can play a major role—but it almost always factors in to some degree. There are various forms of depression, based primarily on duration and severity. The most common forms are *major depression* and *dysthymia.*

- **Major Depression** is what most people think of when they hear the word depression. Major depressive episodes must last at least two weeks, though they typically last quite a bit longer—usually a few months. Major depression involves a significant reduction in the ability to function.

Usually, along with depressed mood, there are physical symptoms like trouble sleeping or waking up, loss of appetite, and perhaps even physical illness.

- **Dysthymia** is similar to major depression, but longer in duration and usually less severe. Typically, people suffering from dysthymia are less impaired than those suffering from major depression. However, it is not uncommon for major depressive episodes to occur in the midst of chronic dysthymia. This is sometimes called *double depression.*

Bipolar Disorder

Bipolar disorder involves both manic and other (usually depressive) episodes. Manic episodes are distinct periods during which there is an abnormally and persistently elevated, expansive, or irritable mood along with increased energy levels and activity. These periods are present for most of the day, every day, for at least a week. Often these manic episodes are followed by depressive episodes that may or may not reach the level of a major depressive episode. Either way, this depression definitely involves a marked decline in mood and/or interest, energy, pleasure, etc. Due to the shift from re-experiencing to numbing reactions that can occur, PTSD symptoms are sometimes erroneously diagnosed as bipolar disorder. A careful diagnosis is needed because they require different treatments. Some individuals may have both disorders simultaneously.

Anxiety

PTSD was formerly identified as an anxiety disorder thanks to the overlap between trauma and anxiety symptoms. However, PTSD is now understood as a more broadly based disorder resulting from stress-related traumatic circumstances. Nevertheless, PTSD and anxiety disorders have much in common. There are numerous anxiety disorders, the most common of which are *generalized anxiety disorder*, *social anxiety disorder*, and *panic disorder.*

- **Generalized Anxiety Disorder** is characterized primarily by excessive anxiety and worry that persists for at least six months and causes significant distress and/or impairment in social, occupational, or other important areas of functioning. The intensity, duration, or frequency of the anxiety and worry is out of proportion to the actual likelihood or impact of the anticipated event.
- **Social Anxiety Disorder** is characterized by fear and anxiety about social interactions and situations that involve the possibility of being scrutinized. These situations may include meeting new people, or situations where the individual might be watched or observed by others. People with social anxiety disorder fear being negatively evaluated, embarrassed, or rejected.
- **Panic Disorder** is the experience of recurrent panic attacks (as discussed in Chapter Two), along with persistent concern/worry about having more panic attacks and/or needing to change one's behaviors in an effort to avoid panic attacks (by not going to unfamiliar places, not talking to unfamiliar people, etc.)

Schizophrenia Spectrum and Other Psychotic Disorders

A wide variety of disorders fall into this category. In general they are characterized by symptoms in one or more of the following domains: delusions, hallucinations, disorganized thinking, and grossly disorganized or abnormal motor behavior (including catatonia).

- **Delusions** are fixed beliefs that do not mesh with reality and are not amenable to change in light of contradictory evidence.
- **Hallucinations** are perception-like experiences that occur without an external stimulus. They may occur in any sen-

sory modality, but auditory hallucinations (hearing voices, usually from outside the self) are the most common.

- **Disorganized Thinking** is typically inferred from an individual's speech, with the person lacking in coherence, switching from one topic to another, and/or answering questions in ways that are either obliquely or completely unrelated to the actual query.
- **Grossly Disorganized or Abnormal Motor Behavior** manifests in any number of ways, ranging from childlike silliness to unspecified agitation to immobilization (catatonia). Often people have trouble performing tasks of daily living.

Addiction and Compulsions

A major connection exists between trauma and addictions of all sorts. Over two-thirds of the people seeking treatment for substance abuse and other forms of addiction also report a history of trauma, often but not always complex trauma in childhood. Substance abusers are two to three times as likely as non-substance abusers to have experienced or witnessed at least one serious incident of trauma. Among men diagnosed with PTSD, alcoholism is the most common co-occurring disorder. Among women diagnosed with PTSD, depression is the most common co-occurring disorder, followed closely by alcoholism.

One large-scale study that measured the relationship between addiction and childhood trauma (including emotional abuse, physical abuse, sexual abuse, neglect, having a mentally ill or addicted parent, losing a parent to divorce or death, living in a house with domestic violence, and having an incarcerated parent) found that compared to a child with no traumatic experiences, a child with four or more traumatic experiences was five times more likely to become an alcoholic and 60% more likely to become obese. Furthermore, a boy with four or more traumatic experiences was a whopping 46 times more likely to become an intravenous drug user. In short, there is no doubt that childhood trauma (and even severe adult trauma) greatly increases the likelihood of substance addiction later in life. Research also reveals a direct correlation between trauma and the incidence of behavioral addictions (gambling, spending, eating, sex, and the like).

Self-Medicating the Pain and Shame

Trauma and the shame it creates are driving factors for isolation, anxiety, depression, low self-esteem, and other issues that can make people to want to "numb out" or "go away." When people consistently and compulsively use potentially addictive substances and/or behaviors as a way to numb themselves and avoid uncomfortable feelings, they are quite likely to qualify as addicts and to experience the negative life consequences that typically result.

> *Joseph grew up in a neglectful, emotionally abusive, alcoholic home. He was told repeatedly by both of his parents that they never wanted a child, and their lives would me more fun without him. When he was ten he started stealing alcohol from his parents' liquor cabinet, which helped to ease the pain of feeling unwanted and unloved. At age 14 he realized he was gay, which, in the small town he grew up in, was simply not acceptable. Feeling "different" and getting no validation regarding his sexual orientation caused Joseph to feel defective and wrong (ashamed) in addition to feeling unwanted and unloved. Before long, he was getting drunk, sneaking out of the house, and looking for love in all the wrong places—typically hooking up with older (usually closeted) gay and/or bisexual men who were only interested in using him for sex. Oftentimes he would steal money from the men's wallets so he could later buy booze and drugs. These experiences temporarily assuaged his pain-*

> *ful emotions, but when they ended he nearly always felt worse. By the time he was 18 he'd become a full-blown alcoholic and drug addict, and he was also addicted to sex.*

In short, Joseph's parents were neglectful and emotionally abusive and he felt different from his peers. As both a young child and a teen he was bombarded with external messages telling him that he was inherently flawed and unworthy of love and belonging. His traumatic upbringing and the resultant shame he felt played in his head almost constantly, and eventually he began to behave in ways (drinking, drugging, being compulsively and indiscriminately sexual) that numbed his pain but reinforced his distorted self-image.

Joseph is hardly alone with his experience. In fact, most addicts experience some form of early-life neglect, abuse, and family dysfunction. Basically, their developmental and dependency needs are not met in childhood and they come to believe that they (rather than their parents, siblings, teachers, and others who should have been providing emotional support and validation) are to blame. They feel as if they are inherently wrong, less than, and not good enough, and their endless litany of negative life experiences serves to reinforce this fact. Simply put, they are people who've been wounded, usually repeatedly, in ways that leave them believing, deep down, that they are unworthy of love, affection, and happiness, and that this will never change no matter how hard they try. And when that's the message bouncing around in a person's head, that person is going to find it very hard to live a wholehearted, joyous life. And very likely he or she will consistently seek out ways to self-medicate his or her emotional and psychological distress, resulting in addiction.

Behavioral (Process) Addictions

Almost everyone understands to some degree what addiction is when it comes to substances like alcohol, nicotine, illicit drugs, and prescription medications. Less easily understood is the concept of behavioral addictions (also known as process addictions). Much of the confusion stems from the fact that behavioral addictions sometimes involve activities that are—for most people, most of the time—healthy and even life-affirming. For instance, eating and sex, two of the most commonly diagnosed behavioral addictions, are absolutely necessary to human existence, as they contribute to survival of both the individual and the species. In fact, these activities are so inherently necessary that our brains are preprogrammed to experience them as pleasurable (as a way to ensure that we at least occasionally engage in them).

Behavioral addiction arises only when people begin to use escapist behaviors compulsively and as a way to cope with life stressors and the pain of underlying psychological conditions such as depression, anxiety, low self-esteem, shame, *and unresolved trauma.* In other words, some people learn to use and abuse otherwise harmless behaviors as a way to escape from life and the problems they have with emotional intimacy. *These are the exact same reasons alcoholics drink and drug addicts use.* Over time, certain behaviors can become the default response to anything and everything, engaged in over and over regardless of the negative life consequences that may ensue—excessive weight gain from an eating disorder, financial woes from gambling, ruined relationships from sex addiction, etc.

The most common behavioral addictions are sexual addiction, love addiction, gambling addiction, and compulsive spending. In today's world, all of these addictions are facilitated by digital technology.

- **Sexual Addiction:** Also known as hypersexuality and sexual compulsivity, sexual addition is a dysfunctional, maladaptive preoccupation with sexual fantasy and behavior, usually involving the obsessive pursuit of non-intimate sex via pornography, compulsive masturbation, and/or objectified partner sex. Online porn addiction, with or without masturbation, is now the most common form of sexual addiction. Research suggests that porn addicts spend at least 11 or 12 hours per week viewing digital porn—sometimes double or even triple that amount. Sex addicts who prefer in-person encounters are equally vulnerable to technology, abusing dating sites and apps, hookup sites and apps, video chat, sexting, and more in their pursuit of escapist sexual activity.

- **Love Addiction:** Similar in many ways to sexual addiction, love addiction is the compulsive search for romantic attachment. In today's world this obsessive search for love is almost entirely digital. Dating sites, text and video chat rooms, hookup apps, and even social media sites can fan the flames of these unhealthy, obsessive relationships.
- **Gambling Addiction:** Also called compulsive gambling, gambling addiction is an uncontrollable urge to gamble despite profound, directly related negative consequences and a desire to quit. Typically, gambling addicts will play whatever game is available, though their preference is fast-paced games like video poker, slots, blackjack, and roulette, where rounds end quickly and there is an immediate opportunity to play again. Digital technology offers these games in abundance. Additionally, online gambling eliminates the need for traveling to a casino, dog track, horse track, or any other betting venue. Instead, gamblers can simply log on to a gambling website or smartphone app—from work, home, or anywhere else—load some funds into their account (using a credit card), and start wagering.
- **Compulsive Spending:** Compulsive spending—also called oniomania, shopping addiction, and compulsive buying disorder—occurs when people spend obsessively despite

the damage this does to their finances and even their relationships. Compulsive spenders lie about and cover up their behavior, and they learn to shop in secret. They buy items they don't need or use or even want, often stashing them in a closet or a storage bin without ever opening the packaging. Sometimes they return things they bought, only to purchase those very same items again at a later date.

Eating Disorders

Trauma-driven eating disorders can manifest as food addiction, anorexia, bulimia/bulimarexia, and binge eating.

- **Food Addiction** is the act of eating compulsively as a way to avoid emotional discomfort, much as alcoholics drink and drug addicts use.
- **Anorexia** is a condition of extreme weight loss caused by self-starvation.
- **Bulimia/Bulimarexia** involves a cycle of binging and purging (self-induced vomiting and/or the abuse of laxatives).
- **Binge Eating** involves the ingestion of large amounts of food, often food that is highly processed. (Many of these foods have recently been identified as addictive.)

Eating disorders are more common in women than men, though they are being increasingly identified in men. An inordinate percentage of women with eating disorders also report a history of childhood sexual abuse. The causative link between the two conditions is not entirely clear, but there is little doubt that they are related to a significant degree. One theory is that trauma, by its very nature, evokes feelings of helplessness and lack of control, whereas self-harming eating disorders offer the opposite. With anorexia, for instance, self-starvation is a powerful form of self-control, a means of controlling what enters the body (perhaps in response to sexual abuse), and possibly a means of punishment and/or self-purification.

Another theory suggests self-harming behaviors like anorexia and bulimia offer escape from painful emotions in the same way as addictive substances and behaviors, thereby serving as a form of dissociation. Of course, as with substance abuse and behavioral addictions, the escapist effects of anorexia and bulimia are only temporary, and after the self-harming activity is ended the individual is very likely to experience tremendous feelings of guilt, shame, and remorse over what she (or he) has done yet again. And usually these feelings merely serve to trigger another round of escapist self-harming activity.

Self-Injury and Suicidality

At best, the negative emotions wrought by trauma are challenging to deal with. At worst, these powerful emotions create unbearable states of being that people are unable to effectively mitigate without resorting to extreme measures, such as substance abuse and behavioral addictions, excessive risk-taking, and deliberate physical self-harm (i.e., cutting, burning, head-banging, overdosing, and even attempts at suicide).

It's relatively easy to comprehend how substance abuse and intensely pleasurable behaviors bring temporary relief from the emotional turmoil caused by complex trauma. Less easily understood is the fact that deliberate physical self-harm can do the same. Although these behaviors are generally directed against the self and regarded as self-destructive, they are actually and paradoxically self-preservative, albeit in ways that are maladaptive and sometimes incredibly unhealthy. In other words, the intention with self-harming behaviors is not to destroy the self (except for actual suicide attempts). Instead, these behaviors are meant to provide temporary relief from unbearable emotional states. Sometimes certain self-harming behaviors can become highly ritualized and compulsive, coming to resemble addictive behaviors.

Many trauma survivors are suicidal and keep suicide as an open option—not because they necessarily want to kill themselves but because doing so provides them with an "out" if things get too bad. On the other hand, many trauma survivors do want to die, and they make active and serious attempts to kill themselves. It is not known how often suicide is the result of unresolved trauma because those statistics are not available. What is known is that suicide may be the final acting out of the "messages of abuse and trauma" and the despair and hopelessness that can follow. If a trauma survivor's emotional pain is simply too much to carry, then suicide may be a means of ending the torment. Unfortunately, like other trauma consequences, suicide is misunderstood, and trauma survivors who make an unsuccessful attempt are often called selfish and self-centered, and shamed for their behavior.

Loss of Personal Meaning and Spirituality

Even when traumatic experience does not result in the conditions and disorders described throughout this chapter (and definitely when traumatic experience does manifest in those ways), survivors may experience a loss of personal meaning and spirituality. In short, traumatic events and experiences can feel, for many people, like an assault on the spirit (i.e., an assault on the "self" or the "soul"). This is especially true in cases of chronic attachment trauma. These deeply wounding interpersonal traumas can, over time, drastically and negatively impact a person's worldview, faith in humankind, religious beliefs, and other spiritual beliefs. The good news is that with proper spirituality-sensitive treatment, trauma survivors who've lost their faith in a higher power can re-develop it, eventually coming to rely on their spiritual connection as a source of comfort and strength during the recovery process (and beyond). Often trauma survivors report, after engaging in the process of healing, that their sense of personal meaning and spiritual connection—once so powerfully diminished—is stronger than ever.

Sleep Disorders

Many trauma survivors experience extreme difficulty with sleep, sleeping fitfully or very little, or having their sleep interrupted by nightmares and night terrors. Lack of sleep can be debilitating to mood, energy, and overall health.

Chapter Five
Healing From Trauma

Treatment Foundations

The first four chapters of this book might cause readers to feel overwhelmed and even a bit hopeless about recovering from the effects of trauma. If so, there is no need for despair because, along with all of the other things that have been learned about trauma over the course of the past several decades, a number of treatment methods have been developed, tested, and proven effective. This chapter provides an overview of these methodologies. Before discussing the various approaches to trauma treatment, however, it is useful to understand a few of the underlying principles, including the need for safety, facing vs. avoiding trauma responses, development of the treatment alliance, and facets of posttraumatic healing.

Safety First

It is a given that trauma survivors simply can't heal from past traumas when they are still being traumatized. As such, risk assessment and safety planning are essential foundations of treatment. This "safety first" principle primarily involves an assessment of current risks, along with the development and implementation of skills that can ensure personal safety in the present. When an individual is actively at risk (i.e., still in an abusive relationship, unable to engage in self-protection, continuing in risk-taking or addictive behaviors), establishing safety may take a great deal of attention and effort.

Generally speaking, safety planning teaches clients to identify cues to danger, to review potential responses, to evaluate alternatives in terms of risks and benefits, and to seek support and take action when appropriate. In other words, safety planning is a process in which clients acquire the skills they need to deal with potentially dangerous and abusive situations and to increasingly keep themselves safe. Applying the safety plan is also a process.

Facing vs. Avoiding

As discussed earlier, many complex trauma survivors use avoidance mechanisms extensively in their attempts to self-regulate and self-soothe their posttraumatic responses. They isolate, they keep secrets, they become people pleasers, they get aggressive, they "numb out" with substances and/or behaviors, they dissociate, they bond with their perpetrators, etc. And while all of these mechanisms can shield trauma survivors from pain, they also prevent the experience, integration, processing, and resolution of traumatic events. In contrast, the core of trauma treatment involves exploring and processing traumatic experiences, memories, and emotions as a way to integrate and resolve them. This means that trauma survivors must engage with traumatic memories rather than avoiding or dissociating from them.

Unsurprisingly, dredging up painful memories can temporarily make symptoms of PTSD, depression, and anxiety worse rather than better and can cause a return to old "tried and true" coping mechanisms. As such, addressing trauma must take place in an environment of safety with a focus on containment and healthy coping skills, including the ability to regulate emotions and to stay sober while doing so. To this end, clients are taught skills that keep them from dissociating and help them to ground themselves in their bodies and remain "present." The therapist also helps clients separate the past from the present and to understand that remembered trauma is not occurring in the moment, even though flashbacks and other re-experiencing symptoms may make it seem as though it is.

The Treatment Alliance

Therapy for trauma and related symptoms requires an informed therapist with whom a "therapeutic alliance" is formed. My colleague Dr. Sandra Bloom has aptly described the building of a therapeutic alliance as "relational healing for relational injury." Typically this alliance develops over time and is based on the trustworthiness and attunement of the therapist, and the client's understanding that *therapist and client are working together* in his or her best interests. Establishing a therapeutic alliance in this way can help to undo a lifetime of mistrust—a major therapeutic advance in and of itself. It also helps in the shifting of avoidant, preoccupied, or disorganized attachment styles toward "earned secure" attachment.

Importantly, this process extends to not just the therapist but to others in the therapeutic environment, starting with the client's peer support group. Residential treatment settings, group treatment settings, twelve step support groups, and other peer support networks let trauma survivors safely discuss their trauma-related issues with supportive, empathetic, and nonjudgmental others, thereby extending their treatment alliance. These survivors learn that they are not alone in what happened to them and in the feelings and self-perceptions they developed, nor are they alone in the maladaptive coping methods they've relied upon. In time, they learn to give as well as take in group recovery settings, working for the benefit of all. Often these secondary treatment alliances are incredibly powerful from a healing standpoint.

Reversing the Downward Spiral

My colleague, Dr. Stephanie Covington, has used a downward spiral that increasingly constricts and tightens as a means of depicting what happens to the unrecovered trauma survivor (and addict) in virtually every aspect of his or her life. The result is less and less freedom, less and less power, less and less control. However, with proper treatment and healing an opposite pattern can develop, with the downward spiral reversing and becoming an upward, increasingly open spiral. As trauma survivors move up the spiral of recovery, the loops widen, opening up their minds, their selves, their emotions, their relationships, and their lives. They experience an ever-growing sensation of freedom, power, and control. No longer are they helpless victims. Instead, they are active participants in their own lives, able to affect and even to control potentially negative outcomes in a positive fashion and to engage with others who are trustworthy and reciprocal. In short, as their lives open up, they find that they are no longer ruled by past traumas.

Resilience and Posttraumatic Growth

It may seem contradictory, but the effects of trauma are not always or only negative. In some cases, the traumatized individual "rises to the challenge" and responds with great resiliency and enhanced coping, and feels stronger as a result. Traumatic events and experiences can turn up positives hidden within negatives—silver linings in dark clouds that are sometimes referred to as *posttraumatic growth*. In short, individuals may find meaning in their traumatic experience, leading to increased resilience and/or changed perspectives that lead to personal insight and growth. For example, a cancer survivor might come to appreciate life more, making changes in lifestyle and working much harder to develop meaningful connections. Many trauma survivors are highly empathetic and spiritual, seemingly miraculous in light of what some of them have endured.

Trauma-Integrated Treatment: Sequenced and Relationship-Based

Trauma-Informed Care

Trauma-Informed Care (TIC) is a philosophy and approach to treatment based on the fact that many (if not most) individuals receiving treatment in the mental health/addiction services system have a history of trauma that relates directly to their present-day distress. For this reason, TIC includes an emphasis on universal screening for trauma at the start of treatment, along with an interweaving of information about trauma and its impact throughout the treatment process.

As opposed to traditional treatment models that focus primarily on symptoms, TIC approaches clients from a position of respect for them as individuals—for their survivor skills, adaptations, personal strengths, and resilience—incorporating a problem solving and skill building approach that emphasizes client control and empowerment. It seeks to reduce the negativity and stigma that often accompanies the treatment of many survivors. Clients are encouraged to actively collaborate on and participate in their treatment as a way to break the pattern of shame and being "done to" (disempowered or victimized) and to establish in its place a pattern of self-efficacy, empowerment, accomplishment, and personal pride. TIC also attends to the client's environment (including personal relationships and home and work life) as part of his or her individualized needs, offering hope for healing and recovery there as well.

Trauma-Focused Treatment

Trauma-Focused Treatment (TFT) is specifically directed at the resolution of trauma in order to alleviate its symptoms. The difference between TFT and TIC is that TFT is a component of TIC, implemented when trauma is an overriding issue for a particular individual. For instance, nearly all substance abusers have a trauma history, but for some that history is much deeper and more powerful than it is for others. Both sets of addicts need TIC, but only one group requires the extra focus on trauma that TFT provides.

Integrated Trauma-Informed Addiction Treatment

It used to be that trauma survivors who entered treatment for addiction were treated for addiction and addiction only, with trauma put on the back burner until sobriety was firmly established. It was believed that until a person got sober, little else could happen on the therapeutic front. And it is easy to see why this approach was taken. After all, if you assume (as most therapists do) that addictions are a maladaptive attempt to self-soothe and self-medicate, and that the basis of trauma-focused psychotherapy is recognizing, experiencing, and processing past and present emotional discomfort, then logic dictates clients can't grow past their emotional challenges (their trauma) while they are simultaneously self-medicating away the resulting anxiety, emotional instability, and depression they experience.

Over the years, I have developed a sequenced model of treatment for addictions coupled with PTSD and Complex PTSD. Built on the three-stage trauma treatment model proposed by Dr. Judith Herman in 1992 and much earlier by Dr. Pierre Janet, it involves stabilizing the client before addressing traumatic memories in any detail. My updated model, integrating addictions treatment, recognizes the interconnected nature of addictions and unresolved trauma and the fact that they often have a negative synergistic impact. In short, this model proposes that if both conditions are not treated concurrently and clients don't heal from both issues simultaneously, they may not heal from either. This thought is well-supported by studies showing that addicts with extensive trauma histories have a much harder time maintaining sobriety than addicts without such histories.

The stages of Integrated Trauma-Informed Addiction Treatment are as follows:

- **Pretreatment (Assessment):** Assessment usually involves several clinical interviews (at the point of initial contact with the program and at the time of admission with nursing, psychiatry, psychology, counseling, and other program staff). Psychological instruments might also be administered by computer or in written format, some of which might be re-administered later as a way to measure the client's progress. Assessment is wide-ranging, including many questions about trauma and other crises in the family or elsewhere, along with questions about relationships, addictions, and symptoms of trauma such as depression, dissociation, and anxiety. Based on the assessment, an individualized treatment plan is developed.
- **Stage One:** This stage is devoted to detox (as needed), abstinence from addictive substances and/or behaviors, and issues of early sobriety. Emphasis is on safety and crisis management, along with extensive education about addiction and trauma and their interaction. Twelve step and other recovery programs are introduced as they relate to sobriety and overall mental and physical health. Residential treatment settings may incorporate a variety of alternative and complementary modalities (meditation, yoga, neuro and biofeedback, acupuncture, expressive therapies, massage, mindfulness stress reduction, animal-assisted therapies, etc.) Once the basics have been covered and the individual has achieved a fair degree of stability and a decreased risk of relapse, he or she is assessed in terms of the

need for Trauma-Focused Treatment (TFT), and a continuing treatment approach is recommended.

- **Stage Two:** This stage is focused on the processing of trauma and its impact through the use of specialized, evidence-based (clinically tested and proven to work) TFT techniques. The goal of this stage is to reintroduce and reintegrate trauma response in doses that are manageable through use of learned coping and emotional modulation skills. The therapist closely monitors the client's responses in order to keep the client in his or her "window of tolerance," helping the client to face and process trauma without becoming overwhelmed. The therapeutic techniques available are first discussed with the client, so that he or she may help to choose one or more that suits his or her specific needs. All of the techniques involve some degree of exposure to what has been avoided/dissociated/suppressed, often resulting in a temporary intensification of distress. Clients are encouraged to discuss their reactions in detail with the therapist, who then offers both emotional support and corrective information when problematic or erroneous interpretations and perceptions are uncovered. Shame, loss, anger, and grief are usually at the forefront during this stage. This emotional and cognitive processing of past traumas and associated memories to the point of changed perceptions and resolution results in the lessening of symptoms and, in turn, an easier time maintaining sobriety and living a more stable and satisfying life.
- **Stage Three:** This stage generally begins after the first 30 to 60 days of treatment (often after an inpatient treatment stay ends). At this point, treatment focuses on the client's newfound ability to make life choices based not on his or her history of trauma and addiction, but on freedom from those bonds and a newly developed sense of self-worth

> and personal empowerment. Clients are encouraged to apply their newfound knowledge and skills to a life of sobriety and safety from additional abuse and trauma. Many life changes may be in order during this stage—developing intimacy, recovering from sexual difficulties, improved parenting, developing new relationships and letting old ones go, discussing past abuse and trauma with perpetrators and others, determining whether to initiate a particular course of action (police report, further disclosure, confrontation, lawsuit, etc.), reestablishing a career or resetting a career path, and more. Twelve step programs can be especially useful as a foundation for these efforts.

Although the treatment stages are presented above in linear format, they are actually rather fluid in application, with clients engaging in the different treatment tasks and moving back and forth between the stages as needed. For example, if a client reports feeling unsafe and overwhelmed during the formal trauma processing that takes place in Stage Two, he or she returns to Stage One's safety planning and skill-building to restabilize and practice skills. Once stabilization and skills are reestablished, the trauma exposure work of Stage Two resumes. Throughout the stages there is planning for backslides and relapse, with setbacks treated as problems to be solved rather than personal failures. At all stages, clients are encouraged to take risks with self-exploration in a safe and supportive environment and to engage in new behaviors based on newly acquired perspectives and skills.

If addicted trauma survivors are struggling with core concepts of healing, or they just can't seem to establish a footing in recovery and sobriety, then either intensive outpatient or inpatient residential treatment may be recommended to jump-start the process. These concentrated programs can last as little as a few weeks or as long as several months. In such settings, addicted trauma survivors are removed from the people, places, and things that initiate or reinforce their trauma and drive their addiction. They are instead surrounded by supportive, empathetic staff members and other patients who are also dealing with painful trauma, deep shame, and debilitating addictions.

Needless to say, every addicted trauma survivor's treatment arc is different. Each person arrives with specific problematic behaviors and a unique background, so each client needs an approach tailored to his or her particular needs. Some will respond best to individual therapy supplemented by group work. Others will do best in group settings, making little progress one-to-one. Still others will struggle utterly until they are physically and emotionally separated from the people, places, and things that have perpetrated trauma on them or that remind them of their trauma.

Commonly Utilized Treatment Modalities

There are more than 100 types of therapy currently in use. Many are general approaches used for a wide variety of disorders, including trauma-related disorders. Several were developed specifically for the treatment of trauma. Oftentimes both general psychotherapeutic approaches and trauma-specific approaches are coupled with alternative modalities like yoga, meditation, neurofeedback, massage, exercise, acupuncture, nutrition and supplements (as needed), animal-assisted therapy, art therapy, self-defense classes, and more. Psychotherapy may also be supplemented with *psychopharmacotherapy*—the use of medications to alleviate the symptoms of psychological disorders, including addictions. It should be noted that psychopharmacological medications do not cure the underlying disorder. Instead, they lessen the symptoms and their negative impact, sometimes making it easier for clients to tolerate things like re-experiencing trauma in therapy sessions. As such, these medications are best used in conjunction with a psychotherapeutic approach (or multiple approaches).

The choice of treatment modality should always take into account the trauma survivor's beliefs, values, and personal preferences. The most commonly used treatment modalities for trauma and related symptoms are described below. They include:

- **ACT (Acceptance and Commitment Therapy):** ACT is a relatively new form of therapy that enhances the client's acceptance of his or her status, followed up with a commitment to action. ACT involves the application of mindfulness strategies and techniques. It teaches people to notice, accept, and embrace their thoughts, feelings, and memories (rather than trying to control them). Then, based on this, the individual can clarify his or her values and develop an action plan for reasonable and positive change.
- **CBT (Cognitive Behavioral Therapy):** CBT looks at what triggers and reinforces actions related to re-experiencing trauma and/or engaging one's addiction, and identifies ways to short-circuit the process. In other words, CBT teaches clients to stop unwanted thoughts and behaviors by thinking about something else or by engaging in some other, healthier behavior such as cleaning the house, reading a book, attending a twelve step recovery meeting, or talking to a loved one.
- **Couples and Family Therapy:** Family and couples therapy sessions are a routine part of addictions treatment. When chronic attachment trauma is involved, these sessions can be expanded to address that. In such cases, the establishment of safety within the family/relationship is the initial focus, with additional treatment geared toward relational healing and the development of intimacy, parenting skills, and the like.
- **CPT (Cognitive Processing Therapy):** CPT is an adaptation of CBT, conducted in written form. In CPT, clients write out

their trauma story, which they then read to the therapist. They go over it carefully so the therapist can provide outside perspective and help to identify any erroneous beliefs or problematic cognitions held by the client. The intent is to short-circuit those beliefs and to replace them with a more realistic assessment of and response to the situation.

- **CR (Cognitive Restructuring):** CR is often used as a part of other therapies, including CBT. CR is a process of learning to identify and dispute maladaptive thoughts and cognitive distortions. This modality uses many strategies, such as guided imagery, thought recording, and Socratic questioning (questioning that is deep, disciplined, systematic, and focused on fundamental issues and problems).
- **DBT (Dialectic Behavior Therapy):** DBT is a behavioral therapy approach based on the belief that behavior change can occur through the acceptance of emotions and consistent practice at managing and regulating them. DBT teaches various methods such as distress tolerance, mindfulness, dialectics (discourse intended to resolve disagreements), emotion regulation, and interpersonal effectiveness. While not specifically developed for trauma treatment, it has widespread applicability.
- **EDP (Experiential Dynamic Psychotherapy):** This is an accelerated from of psychodynamic psychotherapy designed to bring patients directly to the experience of buried feelings, impulses, and emotions, thereby allowing them to understand and overcome their issues.
- **EFTT (Emotion Focused Therapy for Complex Trauma):** EFTT is based on the idea that the therapeutic relationship and the emotional processing of trauma memories are mechanisms of change. Emphasizing access to previously inhibited feelings, the clinician and client work

together to modify maladaptive responses to trauma such as fear, avoidance, and shame. Traumatized clients engage in experiential exercises to simulate confrontation of the perpetrator and change the outcome of the traumatic experience.

- **EMDR (Eye Movement Desensitization and Reprocessing):** EMDR is a mind-body treatment where clients bring to mind painful (traumatic) memories and beliefs about themselves while simultaneously paying attention to an outside stimulus (i.e., moving their eyes back and forth or other forms of bilateral stimulation, called dual attentional focus). This begins a process of adaptive emotional processing that helps the client make associations between memories in order to resolve them. The procedure is repeated until the client's level of distress about the inciting event has diminished. This technique, along with PE, has the most evidence of effectiveness in extinguishing symptoms of PTSD.
- **Emotional Freedom Techniques:** These techniques involve tapping energy points on the body, focusing (brainspotting), or counting while the trauma is being recounted. This dual focus is thought to allow processing, although these techniques are yet to be investigated sufficiently and are considered experimental.
- **Gestalt:** This is another action-based treatment. Clients are engaged in dialogues and other activities to help them free up and resolve emotional impasses.
- **Group Therapy:** Trauma often presents challenges that are best dealt with in group settings (rather than in one-on-one therapy). In fact, addicted complex trauma survivors nearly always require external reinforcement and support if they want to permanently change their patterns of emotional dysregulation and problem behaviors. Therapist

facilitated groups can help these clients see that their problems are not unique, which goes a long way toward reducing the shame associated with trauma, addiction, and other maladaptive coping behaviors. Group therapy is also the ideal place to confront the denial that is integral to maintaining those maladaptive coping mechanisms (especially addictions). Such confrontations are powerful not only for the person being confronted, but for those doing the confronting. As such, everyone present learns how minimization, justification, and rationalization can lead to revictimization and the continuation of damaging behavior patterns. Group members are also able to learn which interventions and coping mechanisms work best based on other members' experience.

- **Hypnosis:** Hypnosis is used in the treatment of trauma to help clients with relaxation and as a tool for self-management. Hypnosis should *not* be used for memory retrieval.
- **MBSR (Mindfulness-Based Stress Reduction):** MBSR is a mindfulness-based program initially conceived of as a way to help people with physical and/or psychological pain. It utilizes meditation, body awareness, yoga, and similar concepts to induce relaxation, stress reduction, and an improved quality of life.
- **MET (Motivation Enhancement Therapy):** MET involves motivational interviewing designed to engage clients in a path of behavioral change. The goal is helping clients increase their personal motivation and achieve goals they have set for themselves (like sobriety for addicts).
- **NET (Narrative Exposure Therapy):** NET was adapted from CBT and other narrative therapies. It involves creating a narrative of the trauma with the goal of transforming fragments of traumatic experience into a coherent story,

which is repeated and corrected with each session until habituation of the event is experienced, thereby reducing related symptoms.

- **PE (Prolonged Exposure Therapy):** PE involves the intentional re-experiencing of traumatic events (in a safe and supportive environment and with relaxation and other skills in place) through remembering and engaging with, rather than avoiding, traumatic memories. Sometimes this technique is referred to as "flooding." PE involves the client's making an audiotape of his or her experience and listening to it repeatedly until it no longer causes distress. This technique, along with EMDR, has the most evidence of effectiveness in extinguishing symptoms of PTSD. *Graduated Exposure* follows a similar strategy, but it is not as direct and the re-experiencing is more gradual.
- **Psychodrama**: This is a specialized group therapy technique that involves the playing out of family roles or other issues, with clients taking part as protagonists, antagonists, and observers/commentators. This acting out of roles and/or events assists with clarifying and resolving past trauma by allowing clients to experience it from a range of perspectives.
- **Psychodynamic Psychotherapy:** This is a form of "depth psychology," which is what most people think of when they picture psychotherapy. The primary focus is to reveal the unconscious content of a client's psyche in an effort to alleviate internal conflict, tension, and emotional discomfort.
- **SE (Somatic Experiencing):** SE attempts to promote awareness of and release of physical tension that remains in the body in the aftermath of trauma. SE recognizes that the survival responses (fight/flight/freeze) are aroused but

are not fully discharged after the traumatic situation has passed, and it finishes the dispersal of the trauma response.

- **SIT (Stress Inoculation Training):** SIT teaches clients ways to address stress and improve resilience. As coping increases, the trauma symptoms may be modified and desensitized.
- **SP (Somatosensory Psychotherapy):** SP is an integrative experiential technique focusing on physical responses to trauma. Clients are encouraged to focus on and learn about their physical responses, and to work with them as a way of understanding and completing the trauma response. This approach puts a less than normal emphasis on talk therapy.

Emotion/Affect Regulation

Regardless of the treatment modality, recovering from trauma is a process of learning to recognize and accept emotions as they happen, to face and integrate them, and to modulate responses. In other words, when triggered by a memory of past trauma, survivors learn to recognize that they are feeling some very powerful emotions, to assess the reality of their situation (to understand that they are reacting to the past rather than an actual threat in the present), and to modulate what they are feeling and how they react (the process of desensitization). This therapeutic work is supported by other strategies such as asking others for support and advice, problem solving, getting regular sleep and nutrition, exercising, and engaging in formalized relaxation through guided imagery, meditation, biofeedback, and the like. Ideally, when trauma survivors become proficient in the various forms of self-regulation, they are able to easily and naturally turn to them in times of distress. Of course, this is not as easy as it sounds. In fact, it takes a great deal of effort and practice. But over time this work is well worth the effort.

- **External Support:** Healthy people rely on attachment relationships for emotional regulation and useful advice. This is an unnatural act for most trauma survivors new to recovery. However, over time, usually starting in therapy, survivors are able to build trust with supportive and empathetic people.
- **Problem Solving:** In addition to response modulation, trauma survivors must learn to problem solve. Simply regulating emotions will not help with avoiding further traumatization. Instead, trauma survivors must learn to be assertive about their needs, boundaries, and rights.
- **Sleep:** Chronic stress and anxiety are exhausting. Even if a trauma survivor is just sitting around, the constant fear of what might happen is utterly draining. Healthy sleep is the best medicine for this type of stress. Most trauma survivors are advised to go to bed and to wake up at the same times every day (eight hours apart) as a way to establish a regular, healthy pattern of sleeping. Sleep strategies (also called "sleep hygiene") are often taught in recovery programs.
- **Nutrition:** Just as healthy sleep patterns are essential to health, so are healthy eating patterns and proper nutrition.
- **Exercise:** Numerous studies have shown that exercise is a great way to relieve stress and depression. Trauma survivors should approach exercise with caution, however, as sometimes an increased heart-rate, sweating, and the like can trigger flashbacks. As such, aerobic exercise is not recommended for all trauma survivors, nor is meditation or yoga. In some cases, modified versions of these techniques may prove helpful.

- **Formalized Relaxation:** Yoga, meditation, visualization, breath-work, biofeedback, and other relaxation techniques can be especially useful, helping trauma survivors to both relax and to ground themselves in the moment. These too must be tailored to the individual's needs and abilities.
- **Abstinence/Moderation with Substances:** Even trauma survivors who are not also addicts need to be careful with addictive substances, including cigarettes. Cigarettes, alcohol, and illicit drugs can all be harmful to the body, causing problems that may increase stress levels. Furthermore, many addictive substances lead to poor decision-making, which can also increase stress levels.

Developing Newer and Healthier Relationship Patterns

As mentioned throughout this book, healthy relationships interrupt the cycle of trauma. In fact, complex trauma survivors can learn to spin this destructive cycle in the opposite direction. Just as unhealthy models of relating are learned and repeated, healthy models of attachment can be learned and practiced. Over time, complex trauma survivors can drastically improve both their self-worth and the quality of their interactions with others. Primarily this involves the development of a wide-ranging and consistently supportive network of people. Individuals comprising this network may include social contacts, work and school relationships, professional relationships, friendships, romantic and sexual relationships, and family relationships.

- **Social Contacts** are relationships built on circumstance. They are built on small-talk. Although they are not emotionally intimate, they are important because they foster a sense of belonging and community.

- **Work and School Relationships** resemble social contacts, but they are confined to very specific circumstances. It is not unusual for work and school relationships to become more important over time, developing into friendships or even romantic interactions.
- **Professional Relationships** may not seem overly important in terms of attachment, but this is actually not the case. The boundaries and contractual nature of these interactions (such as in a therapist-client relationship) can provide safety and reliability, which is very useful in terms of helping traumatized people learn the basics of secure attachment. Mentoring is often a significant component of these relationships.
- **Friendships** usually start out as social contacts or work and school contacts, but based on shared interests and life circumstances they become more important over time. Friendships are relatively unthreatening in nature, and they typically entail little conflict. As such, like professional relationships, they are a great way for traumatized people to learn the basics of secure attachment.
- **Romantic and Sexual Relationships** are, essentially, friendships taken to the level of love and sexual activity. Romantic relationships are "primary" attachment relationships that are every bit as important as family relationships, though sometimes in different ways. Because intimacy requires two people to become heavily involved in each other's lives, there needs to be a great deal of give and take. As such, a secure attachment pattern (where neither person "needs" to isolate, be dependent, or exert control) is imperative to long-term success.
- **Family Relationships** can include family of origin, in-laws, and even "family of choice." Sadly, most people who were traumatized to the point of developing non-secure

> styles of attachment and unhealthy relationship patterns got that way thanks to their families. This does not, however, mean that these relationships are doomed. In fact, complex trauma survivors often, over time and with a great deal of hard work in treatment, learn to forgive those who were neglectful and/or abusive, understanding that those individuals were damaged by their own traumas and were doing the best they could at the time.

Through a considerable amount of hard work in these various domains of relationships, even the most traumatized of people can learn, over time, to interact in healthier ways, breaking old patterns of relating, developing self-worth, and eventually implementing more secure forms of attachment.

Life After Trauma

There is no absolute "cure" for trauma and no "one size fits all" approach to healing. What treatment and recovery do is provide trauma survivors with skills and tools that can reduce trauma's power. In all likelihood, unwanted memories of past traumas will persist to some degree or will recur occasionally even after extensive treatment, but they will not be as triggering and debilitating. Instead, they will become more like memories of normal events. Similarly, trauma survivors (especially the addicted ones) nearly always experience the pull of their unhealthy coping mechanisms, even after years of recovery, but with support and attention to applying learned methods of coping with triggers and emotions the survivor can prevail.

Interestingly, the skills that are learned early in recovery typically become a trauma survivor's go-to coping mechanisms. A lot of people recovering from trauma feel as if their healthy coping mechanisms should "evolve" and become more sophisticated over time. And to a certain extent this does happen. But when the chips are down, when the survivor is hit with a powerful trigger out of the blue, it is almost always the basic skills that save the day.

It is important to point out that recovery from trauma does not happen in a vacuum. Simply put, a large part of recovery is dependent on relationships with other people who are also in recovery. These individuals can be found in therapy settings and various support groups, including twelve step groups (especially if the survivor is simultaneously recovering from addiction). Many trauma survivors also remain in individual, one-to-one therapy, as this venue tends to provide a more directed approach to dealing with the emotions that past traumas continually bring up. Whatever the setting, it helps to have empathetic others who can and will provide support in times of distress and need. The good news is that over time and with the support and guidance of knowledgeable, nonjudgmental, supportive others, any trauma survivor can overcome the debilitating effects of pretty much anything he or she has experienced.

It is my hope that this book supports your understanding of the trauma that has happened to you and the process of recovering from it. As you learn to separate yourself from what happened to you, you will simultaneously find your "self" and increase your self-esteem. As this happens, you will be able to develop affirming and loving relationships as never before. Yes, recovering from trauma takes willingness and a great deal of courage, but the time and effort you put into this process is incredibly worthwhile.

Resource Guide

Finding a Trauma-Informed Therapist

As mentioned several times throughout this book, many psychotherapists are not trained to assess and treat complex trauma in their clients. As such, the link between past trauma and current mental health issues is often either not acknowledged or inadequately addressed. This situation is gradually improving, but traumatized individuals still run the risk of not getting a therapist who fully understands trauma, traumatic reactions, and specialized treatment. The good news is that first-rate trauma treatment is available if you find the right clinician. Psychotherapist referrals for trauma treatment can be obtained through numerous sources, including:

- American Psychological Association, locator.apa.org/
- Anxiety and Depression Association of America, www.adaa.org/netforum/findatherapist
- International Society for the Study of Trauma and Dissociation, www.isst-d.org
- International Society for Traumatic Stress Studies, www.istss.org/source/cliniciandirectory/
- Sidran Institute: Traumatic Stress Education & Advocacy Help Desk, www.sidran.org
- State and local psychological, social work. and counseling associations, looking under trauma specialization

It is important to choose a trauma-informed therapist who is well-versed in treatment methodologies that have proven effective with PTSD and other trauma-driven issues. It is also important that you feel comfortable with that therapist—as if you will be understood and supported, and also challenged when necessary.

There are many designations for counseling professionals: psychiatrist (MD), psychologist (PhD), doctoral or master's level counselor (LPC), licensed clinical social worker (LCSW), pastoral counselor, etc. When you're choosing someone to help you recover from complex trauma, more important than the person's academic degree is whether he or she has specialized training in and knowledge of trauma-driven disorders and treatment.

Before launching yourself into a long-term therapeutic relationship, it is wise to make sure a particular therapist is the right clinician for you. The most important part of your evaluation of a prospective therapist is paying attention to how meeting with that person makes you feel. Do you feel understood? Do you feel like this person has the knowledge and skill set to help you? Do you feel as if the therapist is truly listening to and understanding you? Do you feel as if this person will supportively confront you about behaviors and activities that you know are unhealthy? Etc.

Questions to ask a potential therapist include:

- What professional organizations do you belong to? Are you active in those organizations?
- Do you have any specialized training in trauma therapy? How much?
- Do you understand complex trauma? How do you define it?
- Have you ever treated a complex trauma survivor? How many? If so, what methods do you use, and why? Have

you had specific training and supervision in that method? How long have you practiced it?
- Do you have experience treating common co-occurring conditions (addiction, dissociation, etc.)?
- Do you know how to help me to establish safety in the moment? In the long-run?
- What is your philosophy of psychotherapy and methods of change?

You should also ask questions about the amount of time your treatment may take, the frequency of sessions, cost, and timeframe for payment. Many therapists have written answers to these questions that they will give to you. Either way, you will likely be asked to sign a contract indicating your understanding of and agreement with both the therapy that is being proposed and the business issues involved. Please note that some therapists take insurance and some do not, and some will "slide" their fees based on insurance coverage and your ability to pay. Throughout this process it is important to keep in mind that an exploratory meeting with a therapist does not commit you to ongoing therapy with that person. In fact, you may wish to interview several therapists before making your decision.

Some of your rights:

- You have a right to privacy and confidentiality. Your therapist will let you know the circumstances under which confidentiality can be broken.
- You have a right to sign a release of information, to not do so, or to withdraw a previous release.
- You have a right to question your therapist throughout the process so that you understand what is happening and why.

- You have a right to seek consultation with another therapist. (It is good to discuss this first with your current therapist.)
- You have a right to know that therapists sometimes seek outside consultation on an ongoing or situational basis.
- You have the right to leave therapy at any point, subject to the agreement you made (usually to have one last session prior to leaving in order to discuss or correct any misunderstandings and to have a proper ending.) You are obligated to pay for the sessions you've completed.

Therapist self-disclosure and physical touch are issues to be mindful of. Therapists should not over-disclose in a way that makes you feel uncomfortable or responsible for them and their welfare. Therapists are responsible for their own mental health and well-being. Similarly, physical contact should be limited to a handshake or a supportive touch of the hand, arm, or shoulder, and only with your permission. It is not unusual, because therapy is by nature emotionally intimate, for warm or even romantic feelings to develop. Nevertheless, therapists are obligated to maintain professional boundaries at all times. Sexual contact is expressly forbidden and is grounds for immediate termination by you. Therapists are obligated to work exclusively for the welfare of the client and to "do no harm," and sexual contact has been shown to have very deleterious consequences. You are encouraged to report any sexually inappropriate therapist to the state licensing board and local ethics committee.

Trauma-Related Resources

Websites

- Adult Survivors of Child Abuse (ASCA), www.ascasupport.org
- American Psychological Association, locator.apa.org/
- Anxiety and Depression Association of America, www.adaa.org/netforum/findatherapist
- David Baldwin's Trauma Information Pages, www.trauma-pages.com/support.php
- Dr. Christine Courtois, drchriscourtois.com/home.html
- International Institute for Trauma and Addiction Professionals (IITAP), www.iitap.com
- International Society for the Study of Trauma and Dissociation, www.isst-d.org/default.asp?contentID=1
- International Society for Traumatic Stress Studies, www.istss.org/source/cliniciandirectory/
- Male Survivor: Overcoming Sexual Victimization of Boys & Men, www.malesurvivor.org
- National Institute of Mental Health, www.nimh.nih.gov/index.shtml
- Psychology Self-Help Resources on the Internet, www.psychwww.com/resource/selfhelp.htm
- Recovery from Sexual Abuse: Blog Carnival, www.recoveryfromsexualabuse.blogspot.com
- Sidran Institute: Traumatic Stress Education & Advocacy, www.sidran.org

- Society for the Advancement of Sexual Health, www.sash.net

Books

- *8 Keys to Safe Trauma Recovery: Take-Charge Strategies to Empower Your Healing*, by Babette Rothschild (2010)
- *Childhood Comes First: A Crash Course in Childhood for Adults*, by Ray Helfer (1984)
- *Coping with Trauma: A Guide to Self-Understanding*, by Jon G. Allen (2005)
- *The Courage to Heal: A Guide for Women Survivors of Child Sex Abuse*, by Ellen Bass & Laura Davis (2009)
- *Cutting: Understanding and Overcoming Self-Mutilation*, by Steven Levenkron (1998)
- *Finding Life Beyond Trauma: Using Acceptance and Commitment Therapy to Heal from Post-Traumatic Stress and Trauma-Related Problems*, by Victoria M. Follette, Jacqueline Pistorello & Steven C. Hayes (2007)
- *Finding Sunshine After the Storm: A Workbook for Children Healing from Sexual Abuse*, by Sharon McGee & Curtis Holmes (2008)
- *Growing Beyond Survival: A Self-Help Toolkit for Managing Traumatic Stress (Revised Edition)*, by Elizabeth G. Vermilyea (2013)
- *Healing from Trauma: A Survivor's Guide to Understanding Symptoms and Reclaiming Your Life*, by Jasmin Lee Cori (2008)
- *Healing the Trauma of Abuse: A Women's Workbook*, by Mary Ellen Copeland & Maxine Harris
- *Healing the Trauma of Domestic Violence: A Workbook for Women*, by Mari McCaig & Edward S. Kubany (2004)
- *Healing Trauma: A Pioneering Program for Restoring the Wisdom of Your Body*, by Peter A. Levine (2008)

- *I Can't Get Over It: A Handbook for Trauma Survivors*, by Aphrodite Matsakis (1992)
- *Incest Years After: Learning to Cope Successfully*, by Mary Ann Donaldson (1987)
- *It Happened to Me: A Teen's Guide to Overcoming Sexual Abuse*, by William Lee Carter (2002)
- *Life After Trauma: A Workbook for Healing*, by Dena Rosenbloom & Mary Beth Williams (2010)
- *Mind-Body Workbook for PTSD: A 10-Week Program for Healing After Trauma*, by Stanley H. Block & Carolyn Bryant Block (2010)
- *Opening Up: The Healing Power of Expressing Emotions*, by James W. Pennebaker (1990)
- *Overcoming Childhood Sexual Trauma: A Guide to Breaking Through the Wall of Fear for Practitioners and Survivors*, by Shari Oz & Sarah-Jane Ogiers (2006)
- *The PTSD Workbook: Simple, Effective Techniques for Overcoming Traumatic Stress Symptoms*, by Mary Beth Williams & Soili Poijula (2002)
- *The Rape Recovery Handbook: Step-by-Step Help for Survivors of Sexual Assault*, by Aphrodite Matsakis (2003)
- *Survivor Guilt: A Self-Help Guide*, by Aphrodite Matsakis (1999)
- *Writing for Emotional Balance: A Guided Journal to Help You Manage Overwhelming Emotions*, by Beth Jacobs (2005)
- *Writing to Heal: A Guided Journal for Recovering from Trauma & Emotional Upheaval*, by James W. Pennebaker (2004)
- *Your Surviving Spirit: A Spiritual Workbook for Coping with Trauma*, by Dusty Miller (2003)

Addiction-Related Resources

Websites

- Addiction Treatment, Promises, http://www.promises.com/
- Addiction Treatment, The Ranch, http://www.recoveryranch.com/
- Compulsive Spending, http://www.indiana.edu/~engs/hints/shop.html
- Gambling Addiction, http://www.helpguide.org/mental/gambling_addiction.php
- Love Addiction, The Sexual Recovery Institute, http://www.sexualrecovery.com/
- Sex Addiction, Dr. Patrick Carnes, www.sexhelp.com
- Sex Addiction, The Sexual Recovery Institute, http://www.sexualrecovery.com/
- Sex Addiction and Sexual Health, The Society for the Advancement of Sexual Health, http://sash.net/
- Sex Addiction and Trauma, The International Institute for Trauma & Addiction Professionals, http://www.iitap.com/
- Substance Addiction, The National Council on Alcoholism and Drug Dependence, http://www.ncadd.org/index.php/recovery-support/definition
- Substance Addiction, The National Institute on Drug Abuse, http://www.drugabuse.gov/
- Substance Addiction, The Substance Abuse and Mental Health Services Administration, http://www.samhsa.gov/
- Video game addiction, http://www.video-game-addiction.org/

- Video game addiction, http://www.webmd.com/mental-health/features/video-game-addiction-no-fun

Books

- *Alcoholics Anonymous (Fourth Edition)*, by Alcoholics Anonymous (2002)
- *Always Turned On: Facing Sex Addiction in the Digital Age*, by Robert Weiss & Jennifer Schneider (2014)
- *Bought Out and Spent! Recovery from Compulsive Shopping and Spending*, by Terrence Daryl Schulman (2008)
- *Breaking the Cycle: Free Yourself from Sex Addiction, Porn Obsession, and Shame*, by George Collins & Andrew Adleman (2011)
- *Change Your Gambling, Change Your Life: Strategies for Managing Your Gambling and Improving Your Finances, Relationships, and Health*, by Howard Shaffer, PhD (2012)
- *Contrary to Love: Helping the Sexual Addict*, by Patrick Carnes (1994)
- *Cruise Control: Understanding Sex Addiction in Gay Men (Second Edition)*, by Robert Weiss (2013)
- *Cyber Junkie: Escape the Gaming and Internet Trap*, by Kevin Roberts (2010)
- *Don't Call it Love: Recovery from Sex Addiction*, by Patrick Carnes (1992)
- *Facing Addiction: Starting Recovery from Alcohol and Drugs*, by Patrick Carnes, Stephanie Carnes & John Bailey (2011)
- *Gripped by Gambling*, by Marilyn Lancelot (2007)
- *Hooked on Games: The Lure and Cost of Video Game and Internet Addiction*, by Andrew P Doan, Brooke Strickland & Douglas Gentile (2012)
- *Living Sober*, by Alcoholics Anonymous (2002)
- *Narcotics Anonymous*, by World Services Office (2008)

- *Out of the Shadows: Understanding Sex Addiction*, by Patrick Carnes (2001)
- *Overcoming Your Pathological Gambling: Workbook*, by Robert Ladouceur & Stella Lachance (2006)
- *Pocket Sponsor, 24/7 Back to the Basics Support for Addiction Recovery*, by Shelly Marshall (2007)
- *Spent: Break the Buying Obsession and Discover Your True Worth*, by Sally Palaian (2009)
- *The Me I Want to Be: Becoming God's Best Version of You*, by John Ortberg (2009)
- *To Buy or Not to Buy: Why We Overshop, and How to Stop*, by April Benson (2008)
- *Trauma and the Twelve Steps*, by Jamie Marich (2013)
- *Twelve Steps and Twelve Traditions*, by Alcoholics Anonymous (2002)
- *Twenty Four Hours a Day*, by Anonymous (2013)

Twelve Step Groups

- Alcoholics Anonymous, 212-870-3400, www.aa.org
- Clutterers Anonymous, https://sites.google.com/site/clutterersanonymous/Home?pli=1
- Cocaine Anonymous, 800-347-8998, www.ca.org
- Crystal Meth Anonymous, 855-638-4383, http://www.crystalmeth.org/index.php
- Debtors Anonymous, 800-421-2383, www.debtorsanonymous.org
- Emotions Anonymous, 651-647-9712, www.emotionsanonymous.org
- Emotional Health Anonymous, http://emotionalhealthanonymous.org/

- Food Addicts in Recovery Anonymous, http://www.foodaddicts.org/
- Food Addicts Anonymous, http://www.foodaddictsanonymous.org/
- Gamblers Anonymous, 213-386-8789, www.gamblersanonymous.org
- Heroin Anonymous, http://www.heroin-anonymous.org/
- Marijuana Anonymous, 800-766-6779, www.marijuana-anonymous.org
- Narcotics Anonymous, 818-773-9999, www.na.org
- Nicotine Anonymous, www.nicotine-anonymous.org
- On-Line Gamers Anonymous (OLGA), http://www.olganon.org/
- Overeaters Anonymous, www.oa.org
- Pills Anonymous, http://www.pillsanonymous.org/
- Recoveries Anonymous (RA), http://www.r-a.org/i-video-game-addiction.htm
- Sex Addicts Anonymous, 713-869-4902, www.sexaa.org
- Sex and Love Addicts Anonymous, 210-828-7900, www.slaafws.org
- Sexaholics Anonymous, 866-424-8777, www.sa.org
- Sexual Compulsives Anonymous, 310-859-5585, www.sca-recovery.org
- Spenders Anonymous, http://www.spenders.org/home.html
- Survivors of Incest Anonymous, 410-282-3400, www.siawso.org
- Underearners Anonymous, http://underearnersanonymous.org/
- Workaholics Anonymous, http://www.workaholics-anonymous.org/page.php?page=home

Resources for Partners and Families of Addicts

Websites

- Addiction Treatment Magazine, www.addictiontreatmentmagazine.com/addiction/drug-addiction/how-to-deal-with-your-partners-drug-abuse/
- E-Zine, ezinearticles.com/?Partners-of-Addicts---5-Steps-to-Coping-With-Life-As-the-Partner-of-an-Addict&id=2125557
- Codependency, http://www.nmha.org/go/codependency

Books

- *A Couple's Guide to Sexual Addiction: A Step-by-Step Plan to Rebuild Trust and Restore Intimacy*, by Paldrom Collins & George Collins (2011)
- *Codependents Guide to the Twelve Steps*, by Melody Beattie (1992)
- *Codependent No More: How to Stop Controlling Others and Start Caring for Yourself*, by Melody Beattie (1986)
- *Codependent No More Workbook*, by Melody Beattie (2011)
- *Facing Codependence: What It Is, Where It Comes From, How It Sabotages Our Lives*, by Pia Mellody, Andrea Wells Miller & J. Keith Miller (1989)
- *Mending a Shattered Heart: A Guide to Partners of Sex Addicts*, by Stephanie Carnes (2011)
- *Open Hearts: Renewing Relationships with Recovery, Romance & Reality*, by Patrick Carnes, Debra Laaser & Mark Laaser (1999)
- *Ready to Heal: Breaking Free of Addictive Relationships*, by Kelly McDaniel (2012)
- *Sex, Lies, and Forgiveness (Third Edition)*, Jennifer Schneider & Burt Schneider (2004)

Twelve Step Groups

- Adult Children of Alcoholics, 310-534-1815, www.adultchildren.org
- Al-Anon, 800-344-2666, www.al-anon-alateen.org
- Alateen (ages 12 to 17), 800-356-9996, www.al-anon-alateen.org
- Co-Anon, www.co-anon.org
- Co-Dependents Anonymous, 602-277-7991, www.codependents.org
- Co-Dependents of Sex Addicts (COSA), 612-537-6904, www.cosa-recovery.org
- Families Anonymous, 310-815-8010, www.familiesanonymous.org
- Recovering Couples Anonymous, 314-997-9808, www.recovering-couples.org
- S-Anon, 615-833-3152, www.sanon.org

Other Helpful Books (by Subject)

Anger Management

- *ACT on Life Not on Anger: The New Acceptance & Commitment Therapy Guide to Problem Anger*, by Georg H. Eifert, Matthew McKay, John P. Forsyth & Steven C. Hayes (2006)
- *The Anger Control Workbook*, by Matthew McKay & Peter D. Rogers (2000)
- *The Anger Workbook for Teens: Activities to Help You Deal with Anger and Frustration*, by Raychelle Cassada Lohmann (2009)
- *Daily Meditations for Calming Your Anxious Mind*, by Jeffrey Brantley & Wendy Millstine (2008)

- *Freeing the Angry Mind: How Men Can Use Mindfulness and Reason to Save Their Lives and Relationships*, by C. Peter Bankart & David B. Wexler (2006)
- *The Gift of Anger: Seven Steps to Uncover the Meaning of Anger and Gain Awareness, True Strength, and Peace*, by Marcia Cannon (2011)
- *Letting Go of Anger: The Eleven Most Common Anger Styles and What to Do About Them*, by Ronald Potter-Efron & Patricia Potter-Efron (2006)
- *Transforming Anger: The Heartmath Solution for Letting Go of Rage, Frustration, and Irritation,* by Doc Childre & Deborah Rozman (2003)
- *When Anger Hurts: Quieting the Storm Within*, by Matthew McKay & Peter D. Rogers (2003)

Anxiety

- *The Anxiety and Avoidance Workbook*, by M. A. Tompkins (2012)
- *The Anxiety and Phobia Workbook*, by E. J. Bourne (2011)
- *Client Manual for Overcoming Generalized Anxiety Disorder*, by J. White (1999)
- *The Cognitive Behavioral Workbook for Anxiety*, by B. J. Knaus (2008)
- *Coping with Anxiety: 10 Simple Ways to Relieve Anxiety, Fear &* Worry, by E. J. Bourne (2003)
- *The Dialectical Behavior Therapy Skills Workbook for Anxiety: Breaking Free from Worry, Panic, PTSD, and Other Anxiety Symptoms*, by A. L. Chapman, K. L. Gratz & M. T. Tull (2011)
- *Dying of Embarrassment*, by B. Markway (1992)
- *An End To Panic*, by E. Zuercher-White (1998)
- *The Hidden Faces of Shyness*, by F. Schneier & L. Welkowitz (1996)

- *Mastery of Your Anxiety and Panic: Client Workbook*, by D. Barlow & M. G. Craske (2006)
- *The Mindfulness and Acceptance Workbook for Anxiety*, by J. P. Forsyth & G. H. Eifert
- *Quiet Your Mind and Get to Sleep*, by C. E. Carney & R. Manber (2009)
- *The Worry Trap*, by C. LeJeune (2007)

Depression

- *The Anti-Depressant Survival Program: How to Beat the Side Effects and Enhance the Benefits of Your Medication*, by R. J. Hedeya (2000)
- *The Cognitive Behavioral Workbook for Depression*, by B. J. Knaus & A. Ellis (2006)
- *Control Your Depression*, by P. M. Lewinsohn, R. F. Munoz, M. A. Youngren & A. M. Zeiss (1992)
- *Ending the Depression Cycle*, by P. J. Bieling & M. M. Antony (2003)
- *How To Cope With Depression*, by R. DePaulo & K. Albow (1996)
- *Living Well with Depression & Bipolar Disorder*, by J. McManamy (2006)
- *Unstuck: Your Guide to the Seven-Stage Journey Out of Depression*, by J. S. Gordon (2008)

Dissociation

- *Amongst Ourselves: A Self-Help Guide to Living with Dissociative Identity Disorder*, by T. Alderman & K. Marshall (1998)
- *Coping with Trauma-Related Dissociation: Skills Training for Patients and Therapists*, by S. Boon, C. Steele & O. Van der Hart (2011)
- *The Dissociative Identity Disorder Sourcebook*, by D. B. Haddock (2001)

- *The Effects of DID on Children of Trauma Survivors*, by E. Giller (1995)
- *Got Parts? An Insider's Guide to Managing Life Successfully with Dissociative Identity Disorder*, by ATW & R. Ritter (2005)
- *Mending Ourselves: Expressions of Healing & Self-Integration*, by W. Lynn (1993)
- *The Multiple's Guide to Harmonized Family Living: A Healthy Alternative (or Prelude) to Integration*, by T. Whitman & S. C. Shore (1994)
- *The Stranger in the Mirror*, by M. Steinberg & M. Schnall (2001)

Relationships

- *Allies in Healing: When the Person You Love was Sexually Abused as a Child*, by L. Davis (1991)
- *The Courage to Trust*, by C. L. Wall (2005)
- *Ghosts in the Bedroom: Guide for Partners of Incest Survivors*, by K. Graber (1992)
- *Healing Together: A Couple's Guide to Coping with Trauma and Post-traumatic Stress*, by S. Phillips & D. Kane (2009)
- *If the Man You Love Was Abused: A Couple's Guide to Healing*, by M. H. Browne & M. M. Browne (2007)
- *In Harm's Way: Help for the Wives of Military Men, Police, EMTs, and Firefighters*, by A. Matsakis (2005)
- *I Thought We'd Never Speak Again: The Road from Estrangement to Reconciliation*, by L. Davis (2002)
- *The Mindful Couple: How Acceptance and Mindfulness Can Lead You to the Love You Want*, by R. D. Walser & D. Westrup (2009)
- *Parenting From the Inside Out: How a Deeper Understanding Can Help You Raise Children Who Thrive*, by D. J. Siegel & M. Hartzell (2003)

- *Recreating Your Self: Help for Adult Children of Dysfunctional Families*, by N. J. Napier (1990)
- *The Stop Walking on Eggshells Workbook*, by R. Kreger & J. P. Shirley (2002)
- *Trust after Trauma: A Guide to Relationships for Survivors and Those Who Love Them*, by A. Matsakis (1998)
- *When Anger Hurts Your Kids*, by M. McKay, K. Paleg, P. Fanning & D. Landis (1996)
- *When Anger Hurts Your Relationship*, by M. McKay (2001)

Sexual Issues

- *Beyond Betrayal: Taking Charge of Your Life after Boyhood Sexual* Abuse, by R. B. Gartner (2005)
- *Breaking Free: Help for Survivors of Child Sexual Abuse*, by C. Ainscough & K. Toon (2000)
- *Healing Sex: A Mind-Body Approach to Healing Sexual Trauma*, by S. Haines (2007)
- *How Long Does it Hurt? A Guide to Recovering from Incest and Sexual Abuse for Teenagers, Their Friends, and Their Families*, by E. Gil, C. L. Mather, K. E. Debye & J. Wood (2004)
- *The Porn Trap: The Essential Guide to Overcoming Problems Caused by Pornography*, by W. Maltz & L. Maltz (2008)
- *The Sexual Healing Journey: A Guide for Survivors of Child Sexual Abuse*, by W. Maltz (2001)
- *The Survivors Guide to Sex: How to Have an Empowered Sex Life after Child Sexual Abuse*, by S. Haines (2001)

Author Biography

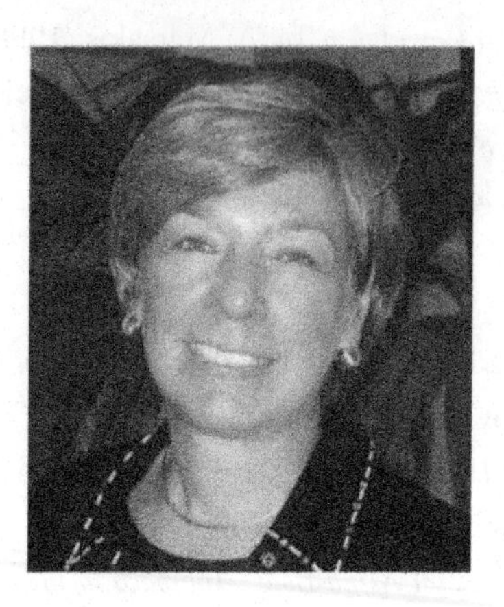

Christine A. Courtois, PhD, ABPP is a Board Certified Counseling Psychologist in independent practice in Washington, DC, and National Clinical Training Consultant for Elements Behavioral Health and Promises, Malibu. She received her PhD from the University of Maryland, College Park in 1979. Dr. Courtois is the author/editor of numerous books, including:

- *Spiritually-Oriented Psychotherapy for Trauma*, coedited with Dr. Donald Walker and Dr. Jamie Aten (2014)
- *Treating Complex Traumatic Stress Disorders in Children and Adolescents*, coedited with Dr. Julian Ford (2013)
- *Treatment of Complex Trauma: A Sequenced, Relationship-Based Approach*, coauthored with Dr. Julian Ford (2012)
- *Healing the Incest Wound: Adult Survivors in Therapy, Second Edition* (2010)

- *Treating Complex Traumatic Stress Disorders: An Evidence-Based Guide*, coedited with Dr. Julian Ford (2009)
- *Recollections of Sexual Abuse: Treatment Principles and Guidelines* (1999)

Dr. Courtois is the appointed chair of the American Psychological Association's PTSD Guideline Development Panel, and has organized the development of guidelines for the treatment of complex trauma for four professional organizations. She is past President of Division 56 (Psychological Trauma) of the APA, and a Founding Associate Editor of the division's journal, *Psychological Trauma: Theory, Research, Practice, & Policy*. In 1990, she cofounded (with Joan Turkus, MD) one of the first inpatient trauma programs in the United States—The CENTER: Posttraumatic Disorders Program—serving as Clinical and Training Director for 16 years.

Dr. Courtois has received the following major professional awards:

- **2010 Print Media Award** (with coeditor Dr. Julian Ford) for *Treating Complex Traumatic Stress Disorders: An Evidence-Based Guide*, International Society for the Study of Trauma and Dissociation
- **2008 Outstanding Alumni Award**, College of Education, Alumni Association, University of Maryland, College Park
- **2007 Alumni Outstanding Professional Award**, College of Education, University of Maryland, College Park
- **2007 Outstanding Contributions to Professional Practice Award**, Division 56 (Psychological Trauma), American Psychological Association
- **2006 Lifetime Achievement Award**, International Society for the Study of Trauma and Dissociation
- **2005 Distinguished Contribution to the Psychology of Women Award**, Committee on the Psychology of Women, American Psychological Association

- **2003 Sarah Haley Award for Clinical Excellence**, International Society for Traumatic Stress Studies
- **2001 Cornelia Wilbur Award**, International Society for the Study of Dissociation
- **1996 Award for Distinguished Contributions to Psychology as a Professional Practice**, American Psychological Association

Elements Behavioral Health and EBH Treatment Facilities

Elements Behavioral Health treatment programs are dedicated to helping clients and their families manage emotional distress and ground themselves in their resilience, across a family of addiction and mental health treatment centers. Our mission is to address the different therapeutic needs of clients within their differing financial means. We partner with clinicians and families in this effort.

Our goal for clients is full recovery and wellbeing with permanent life-change and lifestyle improvement, not just symptom reduction. Our goal is to help create extraordinary lives. For more information please visit us at www.elementsbehavioralhealth.com or call us at 888.627.0772.

PROMISES™

MALIBU, CA & MAR VISTA, CA.

Recovery begins with a promise

For more than 25 years, the Promises® family of programs has offered an individualized, highly effective blend of evidence-based traditional and alternative therapies provided by noted addiction specialists in a safe, nurturing and healing environment.

- LUXURY ADDICTION & MENTAL HEALTH PROGRAM, MALIBU
- PROFESSIONALS TREATMENT PROGRAM, SANTA MONICA
- SUBSTANCE ABUSE & INTIMACY DISORDERS PROGRAM, MALIBU
- YOUNG ADULT TREATMENT, MAR VISTA

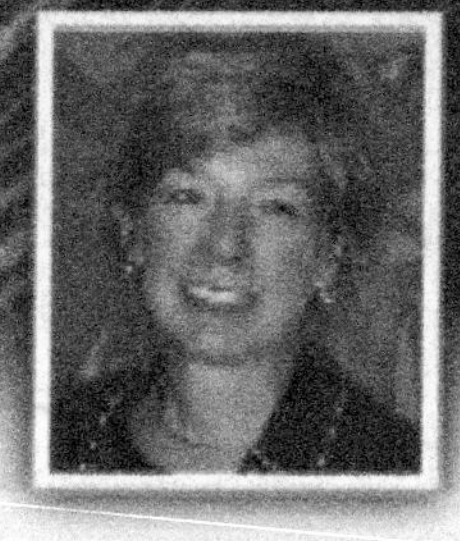

Christine Courtois, PhD, ABPP is a Board Certified Counseling Psychologist and National Clinical Training Consultant for Elements Behavioral Health/ Promises, Malibu and L.A. She specializes in the treatment of trauma, particularly for adults experiencing the effects of childhood incest and other forms of sexual, physical, and emotional abuse.

promises.com

888-901-8854

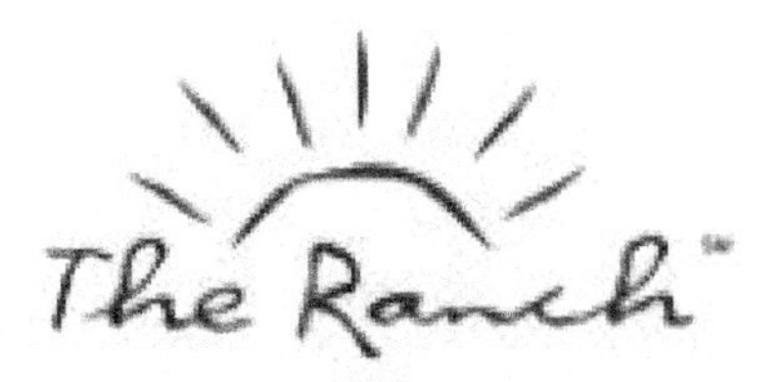

NUNNELLY, TN

Choosing life one day at a time.

Located on a 2,000 acre working horse ranch along the Piney River, The Ranch offers a wide range of therapeutic programs that identify and address both the symptoms and underlying causes of trauma and self-defeating behaviors. Our treatment plans are grounded in a dynamic, experiential model of healing and honor each individual's unique needs and learning style.

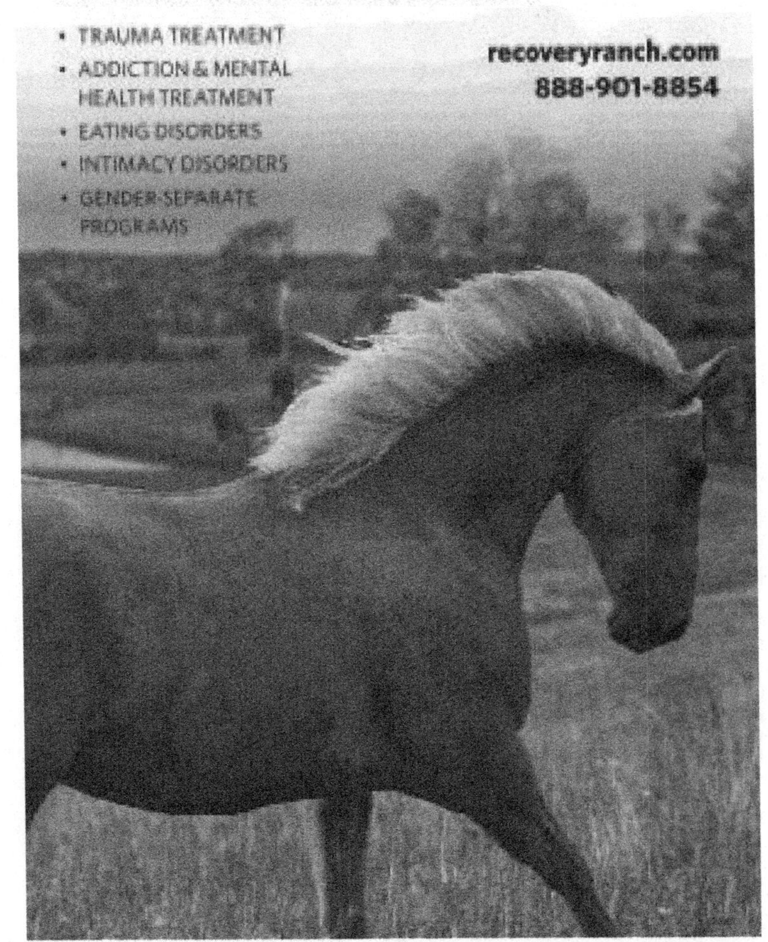

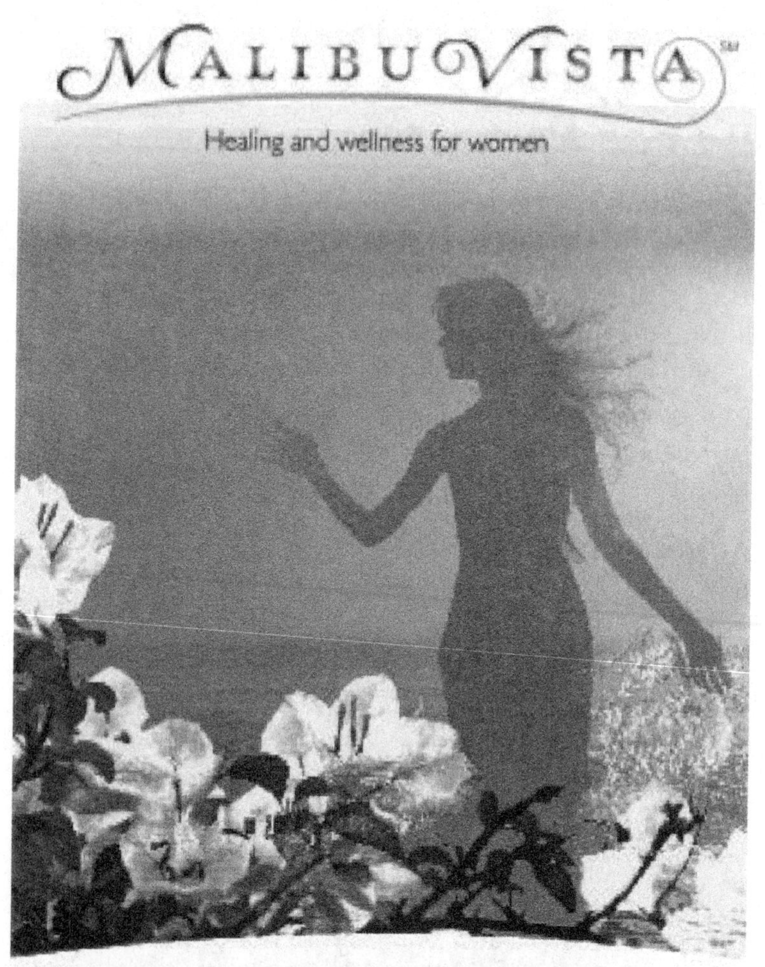

MALIBU, CA — ***Empowerment, resilience and healing.***

Malibu Vista is designed specifically for women suffering from anxiety, depression, trauma, relationship or mid-life transition issues or other mental health conditions. We offer a full spectrum of traditional and alternative therapies designed to help women heal—mind, body and spirit.

- TRAUMA & RELATIONSHIP ISSUES
- MID-LIFE TRANSITIONS
- GRIEF/LOSS

malibuvista.com

888-901-8854

Clarity Way®

Find your path to recovery

HANOVER, PA

Let's get one thing clear: you.

Clarity Way is a leading substance abuse and dual diagnosis treatment center in central Pennsylvania. We offer individualized care and a range of medical and holistic techniques that nurture the whole person to help clear the way for a healthy future.

- LUXURY ADDICTION AND MENTAL HEALTH FACILITY
- EXECUTIVES/PROFESSIONALS OPTIONS
- MEDICAL & HOLISTIC APPROACHES

clarityway.com

888-901-8854

PROMISES
AUSTIN

AUSTIN, TX — ***Excellence is our promise.***

Promises Austin is a Joint Commission accredited addiction and dual diagnosis treatment center for men and women ages 26 and older. Promises Austin is designed for clients who are looking for exceptional holistic treatment in a setting that inspires lasting change.

- LUXURY ADDICTION & MENTAL HEALTH PROGRAM
- TRAUMA-INFORMED CARE
- INTENSIVE FAMILY PROGRAM

promisesaustin.com
888-901-8854

Sundance℠

SCOTTSDALE, AZ

Holistic healing for mind, body & spirit.

At The Sundance Center, holistic addiction treatment isn't a catchphrase. Our program is overseen by a full-time, onsite naturopathic physician and team of master's level clinicians who take a truly integrative approach to health care. We are committed to finding answers to our clients' health concerns, whether those answers come from conventional or non-conventional medicine, so that they can go on to live sober, satisfying lives.

- ADDICTION & MENTAL HEALTH FACILITY
- HOLISTIC APPROACH

sundancecenter.com

888-901-8854

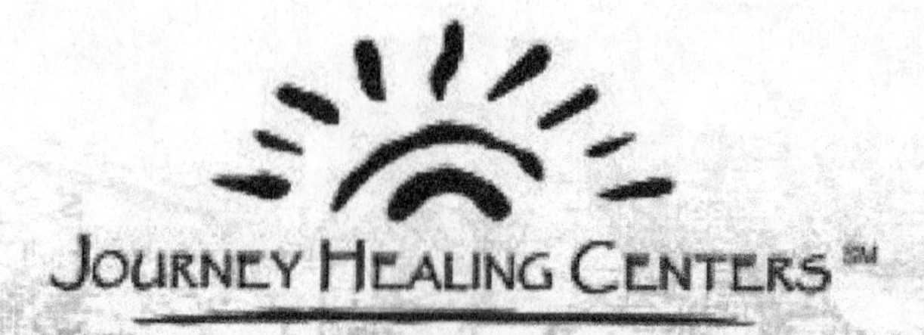

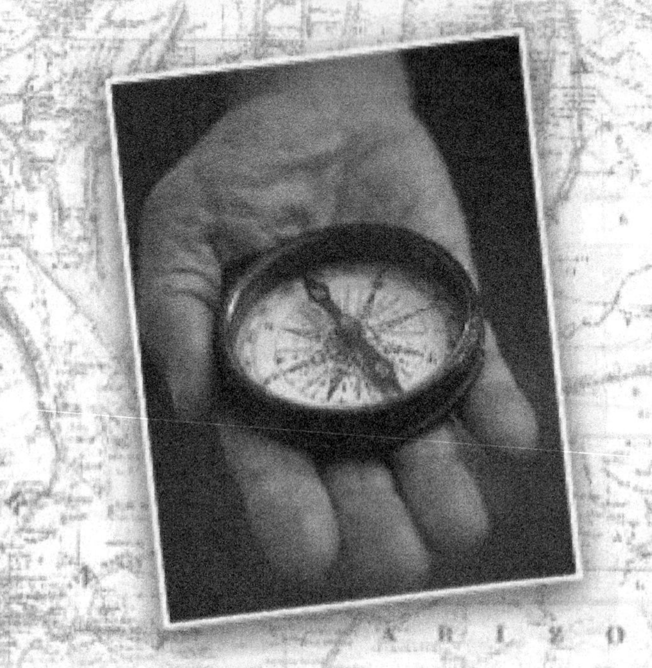

SALT LAKE CITY, UT – ***Change your journey, change your life.***

Journey Healing Center offers an exclusive addiction treatment experience in a serene, restorative setting. Our residential treatment center gives clients the space to embark on a highly customized, holistic care plan while casting off the mental clutter that so often competes with treatment. At Journey, we reintroduce our clients to someone very special — themselves.

- LUXURY ADDICTION & MENTAL HEALTH FACILITY
- CUSTOMIZED TREATMENT PLANS
- FAMILY THERAPY

journeycenters.com
888-901-8854

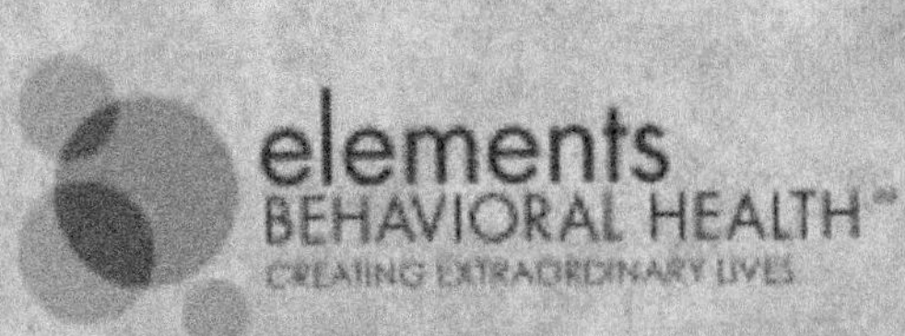

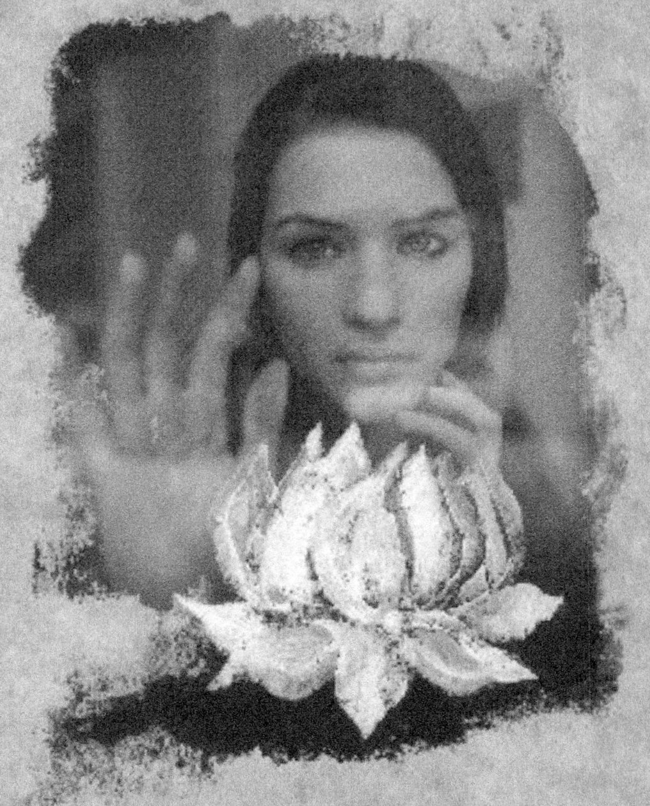

We believe that each life is precious and unique.

We help our clients remember that theirs is too.

elementsfamily.com
888-901-8854